"Dr. Linda is my guardian angel. She has taught me to see myself in an enormously different way. Her work is more important now than ever before because we are disconnected from our bodies, our energy, and our purpose in life. Dr. Linda helps you put all this back together in a simple, old-fashioned way. She reminds you of what you have forgotten, which is what the truly great teachers do."

—Marina Abramovic, performance artist,
author of *Walk Through Walls*

"As I have incorporated Dr. Linda's remedies, baths, diet, and overall care into my daily life, I am experiencing an improvement in every aspect of my health and countenance, most especially the glow of balance."

—Mare Winningham, award-winning actress

"The knowledge in this book paves the way to a new and healthy future for all of us. Part one is nothing less than a state-of-the union address regarding the 'true causes of chronic illness,' which sets it aside from other books currently on the market. Part two could be easily misunderstood as yet another diet or cookbook. However, it transcends all the current—often misguided—diet fads, and the current, rather confused science of nutrition. Instead, Dr. Lancaster reveals simple, affordable, and effective treatment methods, and recipes that are prescriptions for gaining and sustaining true health. I have worked with Dr. Linda for thirty years and respect her as one of the greatest talents in the world of healing of our time."

—Dietrich Klinghardt, MD, PhD,
founder of the Klinghardt Academy

"The connection that Dr. Linda makes between the emotional life and the effects of negative emotions and experiences on the body and overall well-being have affected me deeply. The whole body and spirit are taken into account."

—Anthony Edwards, award-winning actor and director

"Dr. Linda's cleanses have shifted my body, mind, and spirit. She is an icon of healing."

—Gurmukh Khalsa, master Kundalini Yoga teacher

# Harmonic Healing

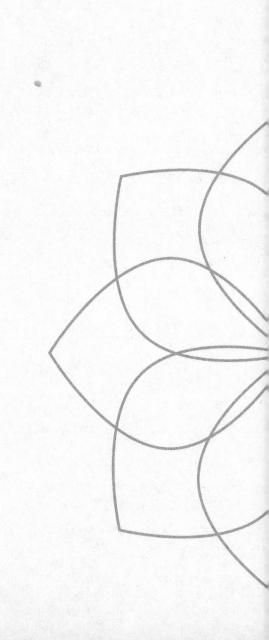

# Harmonic Healing

DR. LINDA LANCASTER

WITH AMELY GREEVEN

RODALE.

NEW YORK

Copyright © 2019 by Light Harmonics, Inc.

All rights reserved.
Published in the United States by Rodale Books, an imprint of the Crown Publishing Group, a division of Penguin Random House LLC, New York.
crownpublishing.com
rodalebooks.com

RODALE and the Plant colophon are registered trademarks of Penguin Random House LLC.

Library of Congress Cataloging-in-Publication Data is available upon request.

ISBN 978-1-63565-317-5
ebook ISBN 978-1-63565-318-2

Printed in the United States of America

Book design by Andrea Lau
Jacket design by Jessie Sayward Bright
Jacket illustration by Macon/Shutterstock

10 9 8 7 6 5 4 3 2 1

First Edition

The energy in the universe is not in the planets or in the protons or neutrons, but in the relationship between them. Not in the particles but in the space between them. Not in the cells of organisms but in the way the cells feed and give feedback to one another. Not in any precise definition of the three persons of the Trinity as much as in the relationship between the Three! This is where all the power for infinite renewal is at work: The loving relationship between them. The infinite love flowing between them. The dance itself.
—*Richard Rohr*

With nature's help, humankind can set into creation
all that is necessary and life sustaining.
—*Hildegard of Bingen*

One can not think well, love well, sleep well if one has not dined well.
—*Virginia Woolf*

*This book is dedicated to my mother,*
*who loved me and my unconventional path in healing, unconditionally.*

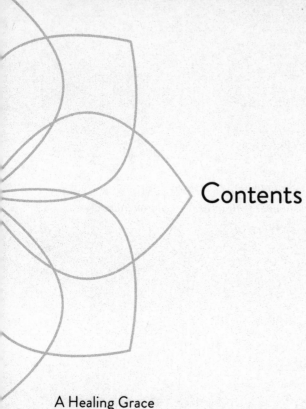

# Contents

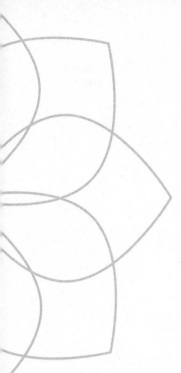

# A Healing Grace

## Terry Tempest Williams

Dr. Linda Lancaster is a global healer. She is direct. She is fierce. She is intuitive and wise. And she is a healing grace upon the planet. Linda Lancaster is a physician who has studied energy medicine with the Masters for decades. She is not only a visionary, but a practitioner who is contributing to a shift in consciousness. I have been one of the beneficiaries of Dr. Linda's brilliance. Quite simply, Dr. Linda has saved my life. My story is one in an anthology of thousands.

If you asked me when we met each other, I could only say, I have never not known Linda. The relationship has been that deep and that essential. I trust her. In the fall of 2009, I was walking out of a movie theater in Ellsworth, Maine, having just seen the film, "Inglorious Bastards." I was troubled by both the violence and the subject matter, the Holocaust. In my attempt to make sense of the film, I turned to a fellow moviegoer to inquire about their thoughts. I couldn't speak. My language was slurred and suddenly, my entire right side of my body went numb. I found my way to the nearest hospital and after a series of tests, I was told I had "an incongruity" in my brain. The incongruity in my brain turned out to be a cavernous hemangioma, a tangle of blood vessels in the Wernike's area of the left cerebral hemisphere. This is the part of the brain where speech is processed, where metaphor lives, and everything I rely on as a writer is located. Hemangioma's bleed. The bleeding causes symptoms such as numbing and compromised speech, in my case. It is also scary. They can burst. The first neurologist I consulted said, "If you were my wife, I would recommend you have the surgery yesterday." He proceeded to describe the surgery, the risks which were sizable including mental deficiency, and the outcome in the best scenario is no more "bleeds."

He was ready to schedule the operation for the next week. I said no. It didn't feel right to me. I thought there must be another alternative. When I gave the neurologist my decision, he said, "How well do you live with uncertainty?" I said, "What else is there?"

A second and third opinion supported my decision to wait and learn to live with this situation until I no longer could regarding a quality of life.

And then, Dr. Linda came into my life. It was at this moment in my life, I learned about subtle energies, the importance of nutrition, cleansing baths, and homeopathic treatments. She also taught me about a more holistic approach to health, in general.

During our consultations and treatments throughout these ten years, she also identified parasites. I have spent considerable time in Africa and this is not uncommon to come home with a sixty-foot tapeworm, which I did several decades ago. So this news did not surprise me. What she said next did. Dr. Lancaster said that she believed the bleeds from my cavernous hemangioma were tied to possible parasites or bacteria in my body. This seemed crazy to me, there was nothing in the so-called medical literature to support this, but I trusted her, and engaged in her famous "milk fast" that consists of taking massive doses of cayenne pepper alongside six glasses of raw milk, goat milk preferably, for eight days, followed by another eight-day follow-up regime of pepsin and more cayenne tablets. I have done this milk fast many times and each time, I have felt cleansed, renewed, and enlivened. My bleeds also became less frequent—instead of one or two a season, they have been reduced to one or two a year.

But here's the interesting part: On May 10, 2017 (several years after Dr. Linda's analysis) the *New York Times* reported under the headline, "A Baffling Brain Defect Is Linked to Gut Bacteria:"

Researchers have traced the cause of a baffling brain disorder to a surprising source: a particular type of bacteria living in the gut.

Scientists increasingly suspect that the body's vast community of bacteria—the microbiome—may play a role in the development of a wide variety of diseases, from obesity to perhaps even autism.

The new study, published on Wednesday in Nature, is among the first to suggest convincingly that these bacteria may initiate disease in seemingly unrelated organs, and in completely unexpected ways.

Researchers "need to be thinking more broadly about the indirect role of the microbiome" in influencing even diseases that have no obvious link to the gut, said Dr. David Relman, professor of microbiology and immunology at Stanford.

The researchers studied hereditary cerebral cavernous malformations—blood-filled bubbles that protrude from veins in the brain and can leak blood or burst at any time.

The findings do not point to a cure, but they do suggest a way to prevent these brain defects in children who inherit a mutated gene that can cause them.

This is just one of the more dramatic examples of what Dr. Linda Lancaster has shown me through the lens of my own body and her work with integrated medicine. There are many ways of knowing. This "great harmonizing" of the body, mind, and spirit through subtle energy work is both revolutionary and practical. I know this through my relationship with the Earth. We are out of balance. The Earth is out of balance. We can work together toward a more peaceful union between our species and the greater community of all beings and find this "Harmonic Healing" by refining our consciousness to be in communion with the Cosmic Body, the Body of Earth, as well as our own.

It is a relief to say this on the page.

The book in your hands, *Harmonic Healing: Restore Your Vital Force for Lifelong Wellness,* may be one of the most important books you will ever read. It will certainly contribute to an awareness of what is possible, and necessary to sustain personal radiance and health. Within these pages, Linda Lancaster shares her philosophy and practice for a life of wholeness carefully woven together through her graceful intelligence.

Gratitude is the word that comes to mind. Because of Dr. Linda, I not only see the world differently, I feel it more fully. Hands on the Earth, eyes toward the heavens, we remember where the source of our power dwells.

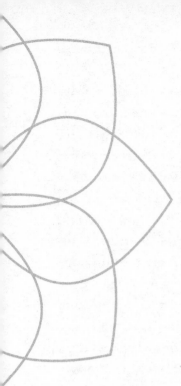

# Gathering the Cords of Knowledge: My Journey with Energy

As a physician, I have always sought to look past the surface to understand what lies beyond. As a natural medicine physician who also works with subtle fields of energy, I have spent a lifetime researching what it means to be healthy. I draw from many traditions—homeopathy, herbs, organic whole foods, cleansing programs, and baths are my cornerstones—yet like a painter who has colors to blend, in the science and art of healing there are many choices.

My journey into the healing power of energy started very young. I was not healthy as a child; the stress of my fractured and abusive home life in the 1950s and '60s in Brooklyn, New York, made me susceptible to parasites that created colitis and depression for years, though I did not understand it at the time. The unstable environment of home spurred me to seek solace in quieter places and ask questions that were beyond my age. *Who am I? Why am I here?* I would ask, seeking help from a source I couldn't name. I found solace at the local convent, where the kind nuns invited me daily after school for prayer, rosary, sanctuary, and relief. There, at age eleven, I discovered that on the other side of all the chaos and noise lay a quiet field of comfort and love. It was my first experience of the peace of subtle energy that suffuses and pervades our material world, and it made me feel safe.

At twenty, like many young people, I decided to set out to make something of myself with a big-city job in Manhattan; but beneath my enthusiastic exterior I was struggling to manage irritable bowel syndrome, which had been diagnosed as spastic colon from early emotional trauma. I soon gave up on the corporate world, feeling called to ground myself in nature. A road trip across Canada and America ensued, and books like *The Greening of America, Autobiography of a Yogi,* and *Siddhartha* were my trusty companions. On my return to the East Coast, I immersed myself in the practice of Raja yoga, which is oriented from the teachings of the ancient Vedic sage Patanjali. In yoga I sought a more direct experience of the harmonious state that had touched me with the kindly nuns, and the practice started to reveal answers to the questions I'd been pursuing for so long. In 1970 I participated in creating a yoga ashram and restaurant on Long Island in what would turn out to be the beginning of an enduring path of yogic practice, and through my study there I received my first energy tool for healing. The breathwork practices of yoga, one of the world's oldest healing sciences, teach about *prana,* the breath of life, in order to strengthen the body, clarify the mind, and steady the emotions. As I practiced the techniques of *pranayama,* I enjoyed a deeper experience of peace and wholeness than I had ever felt before. The breath led me inward to find the space to heal. The word *yoga* comes from Sanskrit and means "to yoke oneself and help unite one to his divine nature." Through yoga I began to realize my self.

Yet it was in the kitchen, not the meditation hall, where I found my personal way to work with subtle energies for healing. It became clear that my fellow yogis could not sustain the yogic experience of oneness on breath and philosophy alone; we had to nourish our physical bodies, which Patanjali called the temple of the soul or *atma.* And so I began a lifelong love affair with preparing and cooking healing food. I was only in my early twenties yet was soon given the job of running the ashram kitchen and its award-winning vegetarian restaurant, which had been founded upon the Vedic principle of *ahimsa* or nonviolence. Cooking with a new level of awareness from yoga, I discovered the sacred power of healthy food; fresh, well-prepared food nourishes not only through its chemical constituents but also through its energy field. I soon found that the foods grown in my back-to-the-land, hippie garden or purchased from the organic farm and sole health-food store on Long Island were the most nourishing.

Intuitively drawing from my half-Italian, half-Jewish heritage, I cooked slowly and lovingly, on low heat to protect the nutrients and ensure ease of digestion. Through Ayurvedic cooking I discovered the healing power of spices. Through working as a chef for *seva,* or yogic service, I also began to counsel my fellow yogis in nutrition. Many of them had been prioritizing meditation over mealtime and shortchanging their bodies by consuming the processed vegetarian foods and meat substitutes that were so popular at the time. To rebuild the weakened body requires food from Mother Earth, not the factory floor: beets for cleaning the liver and gallbladder; leafy greens to heal the lungs; root vegetables to get grounded and mineralize the brain. In Ayurveda, as in many traditional medicines, it is understood that the digestive "fire" is the center point of health, just as the sun is the center of our solar system. By tending to this fire through meals according to their unique constitutions, the yogis returned to *their* nature, of balanced health.

I wanted to deepen my understanding further in order to take responsibility for myself, my family, and my community in a conscious way. These were the pre-Google days; to develop my knowledge of homeopathy, I pored over Hahnemann's *Organon of Medicine* and the *Materia Medica,* the foundational texts of homeopathy, in the wee hours while nursing and rocking my child. Homeopathic remedies are the energetic imprint of a plant or mineral or disease substance that are used to stimulate the vital force to heal; they are based on a system of "likes cure likes," in which one matches the symptoms to those described in the *Materia Medica.* Once a staple in many homes—this medicine was so renowned centuries ago that Thomas Jefferson had his own personal kit—homeopathy was only just beginning its resurgence in the seventies. It carried my family through countless coughs, fevers, and injuries.

Homeopathy took me one step beyond natural medicine into the realm of subtle medicine, and it gave me my first deep insight into how energy holds the key to health.

As my skills developed, I began teaching vegetarian cooking and nutrition classes in my kitchen and basic homeopathy in my living room. Word spread and people started to come to my home, hungry to learn how to naturally heal themselves. By 1981 I had become the director of a holistic health center on Long Island, a new concept in medicine at that time. We integrated acupuncture, chiropractic care, Chinese medicine, and colonics with nutrition and homeopathy in order to customize multidimensional healing programs to our patients' needs. It became clear that our patients were facing a block to well-being that the ancient texts of medicine did not account for: the bombardment of modern-day pollution. Using a new apparatus called a Voll Electro Acupuncture device, I measured the electric charge at acupuncture "ting" points on the body to gain information about what interferences were affecting our patients. Heavy metals, chemicals, radiation, and the resulting presence of parasites were commonly found. It was a breakthrough moment; the device made it possible to assess the energetic body in order to identify the unseen interferences that were blocking the natural state of health.

The people we treated began to get better through this method of diagnosis and the homeopathic detoxification programs that were subsequently given. Yet I longed for a more precise tool to help me navigate the subtle realms of health and to better understand what was happening in the body. After hearing the name of Dr. Hazel Parcells three times in close succession, I took note. Dr. Parcells was a true iconoclast—an unsung hero of energy medicine from Albuquerque, New Mexico. Her pioneering path had not taken a conventional route: When she wasn't seeing clients as a beautician, she was riding on a horse on the Colorado range, smoking cigarettes with the cowboys. At age forty-one she was struck down by tuberculosis with bleeding kidneys. She was told she was going to die and instructed to get her affairs in order. Before she could do that, Dr. Parcells fell into a coma that lasted for nine days. During the coma, she received nine initiations from nine spiritual guides, preparing her to bring the ancient teachings of radiesthesia, a scientific system for measuring etheric energy, to the modern world. Dr. Parcells later told me, "I didn't want to come back with that old body, but they told me if I followed the teachings, I would be healthy and grow to a ripe old age!" Upon awakening, she crawled out of the hospital and began to heal herself through the knowledge she had received about the electromagnetic field. This experience launched her onto a path of deep learning; determined to disseminate this knowledge, she enrolled in chiropractic school and then nutrition, earning a PhD and a commanding knowledge of nutritional science. Dr. Parcells became well known in the field of radiesthesia. She taught practitioners how to measure the electromagnetic energy of the patient at the cellular level and reveal imbalances that led to illness.

Our meeting had its own fate about it. Hesitant to travel to New Mexico since I had a young child at home, I enrolled in a class in New York that taught Dr. Parcells's methods. After the first day of class, I decided that this subtle practice was not for me. But destiny had other plans: That night, I fell into a deep sleep and dreamed of Dr. Parcells's experience during her nine-day coma. Startled by the dream's lucidity, I returned to class the next morning and began asking the instructor such confounding questions that he told me to call Dr. Parcells herself. When we spoke, I recounted my dream, and she told me to come to Albuquerque immediately.

She was eighty-nine years old when we met, vivacious, joyous, and dressed to the nines in Native American jewelry, with red lipstick and dyed strawberry-blond hair, her personal style signatures. She was a force to be reckoned with and I loved her from the get-go. She understood that health is a *process,* not a fixed state, and would famously say when it came to disease, "There is no cure; only pickles are cured! But change the environment and then the condition will no longer exist!" She was the best proof of her own methods: Dr. Parcells practiced in her clinic until she turned one hundred and lived energetically for another six years beyond that doing research.

As I began to use radiesthesia more and more, a broader picture of the root causes behind patients' imbalances could be seen. This method showed the presence of parasites, plus the conditions that allowed them to exist. Radiesthesia reveals how health and disease can begin in the subtle dimensions.

Dr. Parcells was the first of four legendary masters from whom I gathered the cords of knowledge that would ultimately integrate into my own system of Harmonic Healing. As I traveled internationally, teaching radiesthesia as an ambassador for Dr. Parcells's work, I was blessed to become a teaching professor of energy medicine and homeopathy at the Sri Lankan clinic of Professor Anton Jayasuriya, a rheumatologist and master acupuncturist from Colombo, Sri Lanka, and a guru to holistic health practitioners worldwide. Renowned for teaching acupuncture to over thirty thousand practitioners, writing ninety-nine books on integrative therapies, and reportedly treating over 2.5 million patients at his free clinic in the poorest hospital in Colombo, Professor Anton attended to presidents on one day and the poorest of the poor on the next. For over eighteen years, I commuted to Sri Lanka in order to practice at his side. The patients traveled to his free clinic from their villages, barefoot and clad in sarongs, in search of help.

Working at the clinic revealed more insight into the process of disease and that when properly applied, the simplest of healing tools—hands, needles, homeopathy, and breathing techniques—alongside good diet, could release toxins from the body and restore balance to the elements of health. These simple tools had a tremendous effect in strengthening constitutional weaknesses and restoring the patient's vital force and immune system; and they allowed the practitioner to treat the whole person as a harmony of physical, mental, emotional, and spiritual aspects. My years of working with Professor Anton gave me not only new modalities for healing but also an understanding that the most important person in the clinic is the patient. From him I learned that compassion and love were the tools that no practitioner could be without.

At a medical conference in the steamy city of Chennai in the south of India in the early nineties, I met my third mentor. A revered figure in Ayurvedic medicine and an expert in homeopathy, teletherapy, dowsing, and gem therapy, Dr. A. K. Bhattacharya sat down next to me at the podium. I knew who he was, for I had read his books. When Professor Anton introduced me as an admirer of his work and a practitioner of radiesthesia, Dr. Bhattacharya turned his head, took me in for a moment, and declared with no forewarning, "You must come to my home in Calcutta to study with me, and I will remind you of what you already know." It is safe to say that nobody I had met before could match Bhattacharya's sheer breadth and depth of Ayurvedic knowledge. He taught me how to incorporate healing with gems, which in India correlates with astrology, and to send treatment from a distance using a method called teletherapy. Bhattacharya followed in the footsteps of his father, the renowned Dr. Benoytosh Bhattacharya, with his expertise in Tridosha Theory—homeopathy according to the three *doshas,* the constitutional elements of the body. He taught me Tridosha in homeopathy and the subtle science of reading the patient's life force and organ strength with no more than three fingers on the pulse. These modalities became the foundation of the Light Harmonics system that is practiced and taught today.

In India and Sri Lanka, I was a woman in a man's world. The respected doctors of homeopathy and Ayurveda, as well as the astrologers who were considered equally important in healing, were mostly men a stark contrast to the United States, where most of my colleagues studying healing in the new-age therapies were women. I was blessed that my teachers treated me with honor on my unconventional path. Battacharya told me with absolute conviction, "You have original knowledge. Do not read any books for the next ten years. Just write what you know and speak the truth as you know it to be." I followed his advice, learning to speak and teach from my own knowledge and observation in clinical practice.

From that point, the pieces of the puzzle began to fall into place. I began to combine the diagnostic tools of energy measurement with knowledge of yoga, Ayurveda, traditional Chinese medicine, constitutional homeopathy and miasmatic (inherited weakness) practice, and my interpretation of the spiritual aspects of illness and health. In the early 1990s, my family and I moved our home and clinic to Santa Fe, New Mexico, to be closer to Dr. Parcells in her last years, and it was there that my fourth mentor entered my life. Yogi Bhajan, the world-renowned yogi who brought Kundalini yoga to the west and the founder of the 3HO Foundation (happy, healthy, holy) lived nearby on his pristine ashram in Española, New Mexico. Yogi Bhajan was a White Mahan Tantric Master. He brought this practice to the West and worked tirelessly to teach it to promote peace in the world. Hearing of my work, he summoned me to perform an analysis of his health. I dressed in white out of respect for the Sikh culture and arrived to a greeting of "Good. You were in my astrology today. Now you are finally here."

Yogi Bhajan was a magnetic man with a ferocious bark, yet we had a special rapport. Many a night, we would talk for hours over dinner about health, homeopathy, healing, and energy. He loved talking about food! I spent some months cooking for him and teaching others to continue in my simple way of preparing food. For the next eight years, I continued to attend to Yogi Ji, as I came to affectionately call him, as his homeopathic doctor in charge of all the integrative therapies and natural medicines given to him. He had undergone several heart bypass surgeries prior to our meeting, and he was a diabetic; as a consequence, his doctors had deemed him unable to travel. I modified his diet—while utilizing homeopathics to manage his diabetes and strengthen his kidneys. Yogi Ji became strong enough to continue to teach and travel to India again, something his doctors had said could never happen. He managed to return to his homeland twice more before his passing.

Yogi Bhajan gifted me a deeper understanding of the ether, the subtle element that is the space out of which the elements evolve and is the energy that healers use to heal. When I checked his Ayurvedic pulse with my fingertips, he was also teaching *me;* as our breaths entrained, he allowed direct absorption of his teaching of Sat Nam Rasayan—a yogic healing science of pure meditative absorption in the divine that translates as "deep relaxation in the true identity of the soul." I could feel the energy move around his body, moving through stagnation through pure grace. From Yogi Bhajan was born my knowing that in healing, sometimes a connection is all it takes. A word, touch, or a simple presence will in some cases suffice for a block to soften and for space to be created for the life force to return. My experience with Yogi Ji, whom I tended to until his last breaths, was a teaching in trust in the body's ability to heal itself and, ultimately, to consciously let go.

The knowledge of these four great masters, and the lineage of subtle sciences they represented for me, has harmonized into my own system for healing and teaching energy medicine. This system recognizes that in healing, nothing is separate: the physical body *and* the subtle realms of vitality, emotions, thought, and spirit constitute who we are, and for health to exist, they need to be in harmony. It also recognizes how our etheric energy is the way into balancing and healing these realms.

When I started practicing professionally in 1981, viruses were prominent, AIDS was an epidemic, and immune-system disorders were common. Chemicals had become quietly widespread in foods, homes, and workplaces, creating new levels of fatigue and mysterious symptoms, and organically grown food was not the norm. Today we face new kinds of mysterious syndromes—like Lyme disease, chemical sensitivities, adrenal exhaustion, hypothyroidism, autoimmune diseases, autism, Alzheimer's, stress and brain imbalances, and more—that affect a wide spectrum of people, from the youngest to the oldest. The assaults on the energy body have become more complex, and pollution now includes electrosmog from technology's electromagnetic fields that we live amid, day and night.

But while the environment we live in has changed, and the conditions in the body have morphed in response, my approach has remained consistent. Harmonic Healing involves learning to live amid the challenges we face as best as we can, and it follows a philosophy of treating the person, not the disease, encouraging their body to engage in the process of health by creating the conditions for health to exist. It involves helping the patient not only to feel better in their body (by resolving physical symptoms) but also to ask the questions that challenged me many years ago in the Brooklyn convent: *Why am I here? What is getting in the way of my true purpose?* With time and patience, healing can peel away the layers that cloud the light of our truest selves, allowing the light to radiate.

Yogi Bhajan once said that as a physician, I was a hundred years ahead of my time. Time must have sped up, because today the energy medicine that was once considered "out there" is now embraced and honored. Yoga and acupuncture are everyday activities for many, essential oils and crystals are commonplace, and sound healing and shamanism are no longer fringe. My specialty, homeopathy, is a household word. It is a new world order, in which one in three young people say they meditate and the simple action of finding healing in nature, with feet on the ground and face to the sky, is finally understood for the medicine it is. More people are thinking about their well-being, whether they seek to clear environmental pollution before conceiving a child, find invisible causes of disturbance in body or mind, or avoid illnesses they suspect may be possible due to inherited traits.

This great harmonizing is occurring among practitioners too. The equivalent of an interfaith movement is growing as diverse practitioners come together to share knowledge like never before, united by the connection to the subtle energy that pervades, connects, and sustains all life and the commitment to integrate the physical and subtle sides of health. Though the pressure and intensity of this moment is undeniable, the opportunity for growth and transformation is extraordinary.

The medicines I use today are what they always have been: a harmony of good food to nourish the vitality, conscious breathing and meditation to create peace and resolve blocks, herbs to help the body rebalance and detoxify, and homeopathy to encourage the shifts that can occur when the space is open for us to discover who we are. These subtle medicines and the lifestyle they offer have a tremendous potential. They can help us to feel and function better, and to access the space of healing in which the body's natural intelligence is ready to do its best work. They can help us move from where we've become stuck to where we are capable of going and growing. This may sound like a stretch, but it is really quite straightforward. When vital energy is allowed to flow, and the will is reignited and sustained, we feel empowered to reach for the life we want. Our life begins to flow! That is the beauty of Harmonic Healing, and it is available to everyone. I invite you to take your first steps into the space of your potential.

# How to Use This Book

n this approach, which is anchored in Ayurveda, yoga, energy medicine, homeopathy, and nutrition, we look at balancing the energy. I invite you to pause from the busyness that surrounds so much of getting and staying well today. Together we are going to look at your body and your health through new eyes to help you to start feeling better.

The information that follows will be familiar if you already follow a path of natural self-care, for example if you choose certain fresh foods to pick yourself up when you don't feel well, have a favorite herbal tea or tincture when you feel stressed, or use yoga or meditation as a way to find clarity or peace. Subtle energy healing will line up with what you already know to be true—and it may excite and inspire you, because it will open up a broader understanding of why the things you already like to do affect you for the good and of how to make them work even better.

If this lifestyle is not your norm, what follows may be inspiring, but for different reasons. It will show you how small choices each day can have significant effects, for reasons you may not fully have considered until now. Some of the simplest things available have healing potential because of the compounds they contain and *also* because of the quality of their energy field. Seen through this integrative lens, a vibrant apple grown in clean soil can be the medicine that nature intended—it has the healing energy that helps your gallbladder to do its job. And a bath with sea salt and baking soda can neutralize radiation from a day in front of the computer or a long airplane flight.

How do you arrive at this new approach to natural living? In Part One you will be introduced to the different subtle energy fields and the nearly infinite ways in which they are intertwined. This will help you to see yourself in a new light—as a multidimensional being. Then you'll look at how these subtle energies are affected by the environment you live in, influenced by unseen forces that have the power to create the conditions of health or dis-ease. You will then begin to look at the possibilities in play for what is creating many of the symptoms you may be experiencing, and all the possibilities for what can help them to get better.

In Part Two you will learn the protocols for caring for yourself from this subtle level of energy. This launches with the six-week Harmonic Healing Program for destressing the liver and neutralizing pollution in the body. It includes therapeutic detoxifying baths and a dietary program that allows your digestive and detoxification system to recover so that your body can function more optimally. As I share methods of preparing meals on this program that allow you to more easily digest food, you will take a journey into conscious nutrition. This leads into information for *sustaining* this newly revitalized and balanced state through a lifestyle in which an awareness of energy guides your choices daily. The world we live in is not going to change anytime soon; pivotal to the "harmonic" way is that this is a continuum of care, not a once-a-year event!

Subtle energy may seem a bit esoteric, because it is not something we can detect easily with our senses. Seeing the energy visually takes mastery, and even connecting to it takes time, as it is a nonphysical energy. We experience the *result* of energy through our senses, for example as the force of a physical blow on our body, the movement of a breeze on our skin, or the dance of light on our retinas. But should we ask where this energy comes from, the answer may feel a little out of reach. In traditional, older lineages of medicine, healers and physicians are interested in the movement and quality of the life-giving subtle energies through the body; to interpret these, we use both science and art. (Hence the term "the healing arts.") As you read through the pages that follow, I invite you to allow yourself some freedom: Do not try to master the subject of energy and the invisible forces of nature with your intellect. Even master physicists are still grappling with precise definitions of subtle energy, and many of the concepts we hold to be truths are, in fact, working theories. An abstract relationship with energy is not what we seek here; an intimate relationship is! What matters when it comes to energy is not the mental grasp of what it *is* but the awareness of what it *does* and how your choices and environment affect its ability to enliven you.

If you hold only a single concept of subtle energy to heart, hold this one: Health and harmony in the body and mind *begin* at the level of subtle energy. Like the intention before the manifestation, subtle energy is the fabric from which the physical arises. When your awareness holds this, good choices become a little easier to make. The vibrant nature of a food at the market catches your attention and simply feels good to you—it resonates with you at an energetic level—and you know what to have for dinner. (The resonance of a food can also do the opposite—give you a sense that it is to be avoided!) Or you notice a subtle level of depletion in your body after a work trip and choose to take a detoxifying bath rather than reach for a third cup of coffee. Over time, living with this awareness becomes second nature and you make headway into a conscious lifestyle of good choices that support both your physical and energetic body.

Gaining awareness of the subtle is a process—it settles in gently like leaves falling to the earth in autumn or snow falling in winter. Take that first slow, conscious breath—inhale, pause briefly, then exhale. In that pause between the inhale and the exhale is a stillness that is pure potential, consciousness. It's there we can find an opening into an awareness of subtle energy, the receiving and the giving out of life, and it is there that we can begin to heal.

# THE FIVE PRINCIPLES OF HARMONIC HEALING

1. The human body has an innate ability to heal. This comes from our vital force, the subtle energy that we were born with.

........................

2. The human body's subtle energy fields can either be strengthened or weakened depending on the electro-magnetic environment of the cells.

........................

3. When the environment at the cellular level is weak, parasites can take over and become a root cause of disease.

........................

4. When parasites/environmental stress is neutralized, the digestive power can repair, and therefore the vital force can flow.

........................

5. When the vital force becomes strong again, the disease process can begin to resolve.

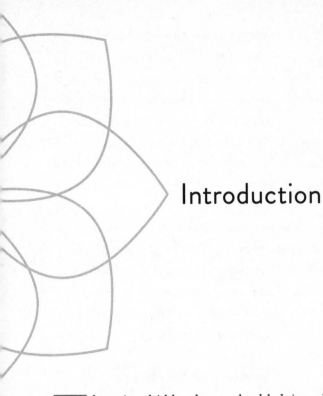

# Introduction

There is a hidden key to health lying close within reach. It is the knowledge that unlocks our body's innate ability to heal, and it is so fundamental that it has long been considered the starting point for wellness. But because it lies just past the normal line of sight when it comes to health, it has gotten lost and overlooked.

This key is the power of our body's vital force to heal. When we learn to access and care for it, we switch on our body's ability to stay well in a world of challenging forces and help our body to heal when we are sick. This force exists within everyone, no matter their age, current health concerns, or predispositions. It's just not as obvious as other resources—like the power of speech or the force in our emotions!—because it lies in the realm of the subtle; at the level of energy.

I have been a natural physician working at the level of energy for almost forty years. I have integrated many modalities of East and West, been a grateful student of the greatest healers of my time, and woven together threads from the subtle medicines of long ago into my own system of medicine that opens the gateways to help the body heal itself. I have been asked to write about this knowledge many times and have always responded that one day, when the tide of patients slowed down, I would.

But the tide has not slowed; it has gotten more swift and pressing, with once-occasional complaints of low energy, digestive distress, chronic pain, anxiety, insomnia, headaches, skin issues, and depression now the norm, and happening at earlier ages than before. Sometimes my patients have seen many practitioners and tried many treatments in the quest to regain their energy and joie de vivre, yet the state of vitality they seek eludes them.

It's time to change course and to share the secrets of subtle energy. Though the patient typically experiences the symptoms as physical ones, the root cause very often is found beyond the physical body. I see it as an energetic blockage that can create an environment for illness patterns to emerge and sometimes to persist. Harmonic Healing draws from integrated approaches and modalities that include the physical and the energetics of subtle medicines.

For almost four decades, I have worked with patients to restore and care for their well-being in accordance with their own individual constitutions and situations. While I offer a personalized approach, I notice some commonalities.

- A digestive system that is not absorbing enough nourishment from food, and simultaneously organs of detoxification that are congested, creating a low-functioning system with low energy.

- Pollution in the form of heavy metals, chemicals, and radiations that create agitation at the cellular level, collectively causing an imbalance in the body's life-sustaining energy.

Each of these factors individually can contribute to low energy, weakened health, and loss of joy and will. Together they can create the ideal environment for parasites—a group of organisms that includes fungi, microscopic parasites, viruses, bacteria, and worms—to grow. These are present in most of the patients I have evaluated over the years. When these parasites exist in a disturbed environment, they can create a perfect storm and become the root of chronic conditions and mystery illnesses.

Pollution and parasites often exist together in layers, with the pollution allowing the parasites to dig in deeper. They may have been there for years, slowly disturbing the environment, until a triggering event like stress, injury, shock, or trauma tips the balance and suddenly the parasites take over. Their effect can be sudden or subtle, sapping the vital energy, and over time these parasites can become layers of a spiral that can pull our health downward. Because it's a *spiral,* it is not the typical causal relationship that modern-day science and medicine can condition us to expect. Challenged to find clear answers to our problems, we can slide further down the spiral, which only tires us further and can interfere with our will to heal. And until we start to evaluate the unseen causes— the body's energy level and the conditions of the subtle environment—it can be arduous, and sometimes impossible, to feel better. The expensive supplements cannot work, the well-intentioned weight-loss programs will frustrate, and the persistent, disturbing symptoms will not get the support they need to clear.

I let my patients know that none of this means they aren't caring about their body or trying hard enough to be healthy! It is a result of our new reality in which invisible forces of pollution, radiation, and mental and emotional stress bombard us every day, while food has lost much of its energetic healing potential. I tell them that *there is a way through this.* Wherever they are on the spectrum of health or illness, I ask them to reevaluate supplements they may be taking, to press pause on any radical solutions they may be trying on their own, and to take a breath. We are going to go back to nature—back to *their* nature as an energetic being!— and start a process of getting their vitality back. We will gently neutralize the toxic interferences that have accumulated over time, clear the liver of congestion and restore their body's digestive power, and fill their diet with foods that are naturally high in vitality. In so doing, they will start to cleanse the body of pollution, nourish their subtle energy, and restore their innate ability to heal.

Their tools in this endeavor? This can be surprising for some, for the remedies will be simple, natural products that are available at stores and markets in their neighborhood. Foods with healing potential like extra-virgin olive oil, vegetables and fruits, good-quality protein, and healing herbs and spices; heavy pots for slow and low-heat cooking, and old-fashioned household ingredients like sea salt, baking soda, Clorox, and apple cider vinegar for detoxifying baths. Even coffee makes the cut: a cup a day is perfectly acceptable in the quest to return to balance.

Though some people wonder at their healing program's stripped-down approach—there are no fancy powders or pricey pills in their bag as they leave their first session—many feel the ignition of an ember of hope (and a quiver of delight that coffee is not forbidden!). They have identified some depletions, stressors, and interferences that they may have quietly sensed for some time but not quite had words for; they've learned that these challenging influences can be neutralized and their well-being improved through uncomplicated, time-tested methods. Shopping list in hand, they go home to take the first steps of what can become a whole new lifestyle.

You might feel like you have been doing everything right—exercising daily, meditating regularly, and taking your vitamins—but not feeling as good as you want. You might have tried multiple diets and put a lot of effort into fine-tuning your food but still feel bloated or heavy, struggling with gas or constipation, or overly tired after you eat. Perhaps, like many, you feel confounded by a mysterious syndrome that nobody can name or general poor health that has taken too much of your time to figure out or prevented you from even holding down a job.

Or perhaps you are simply seeking to keep you and your family's health on an even keel in a confusing landscape of polluting stressors that seem to be getting worse by the year. If you're asking, *How do I stay healthy in this unhealthy world?* you are not alone.

The solution is to connect to the vital force and nourish yourself with etheric energy from Mother Nature, who gives us our potential to radiate in health.

Over the course of a career that has taken me around the globe many times, sitting at the feet of masters, I have come to an understanding that health and the healing potential come from the balance of one's vital force. Acknowledged for millennia in medicines around the world as *chi* or *prana,* it is universally revered as the origin of health and our connection to universal energy. The vital force does not show up in lab tests and it rarely gets mentioned at a doctor's office; it exists beyond the limits of most people's perception and understanding. Yet it is the primary factor in how well or poorly you feel, how gently you age, and how you recover from injury because it is the *prephysical* realm of life—the source from which health springs and where the seeds of disease are sown.

While the vital force exists to give you life, *your* part is to care for it, nourish it, and keep it in balance. Especially today, when balance is becoming increasingly challenging to sustain. You can do this, quite simply, by living in accordance with nature, as the ancient wisdoms taught, and maintaining the organs and systems of the body through simple protocols of nutrition and detoxification, and homeopathic and alchemical remedies to stimulate the vital force as needed.

When I teach patients and students to nourish their subtle energy through gentle protocols, they begin to experience the gateways to increased vitality and better health opening within. When we neutralize the heavy metals and chemicals that have been suppressing their vital force, and the effects of radiation that have been aggravating it, the digestive system begins to assimilate food and patients supply their body with the energy it has been missing. Supported with new vitality, they can start the process of a deeper clearing-out, pushing back against the presence of one or more of the parasites that may have been weakening their health. Because subtle energy is the conduit that connects every part of who we are, encouraging it to flow can begin to release unhealthy patterns that may be disrupting the balance in body, mind, and spirit. Most important of all, a *will for life* is ignited. This, as you will discover in the pages that follow, allows the body's innate knowledge of the vital force to heal. This is accomplished by freeing the liver of congestion, for the liver is directly connected to the mental will and how we think. Taken together, these steps are the foundation of Harmonic Healing.

None of this happens overnight. While it takes time to unwind what has often taken years to create, the energy begins to be restored through neutralizing environmental pollution and eating food imbued with energy. Man and nature are one, and through nature we nourish ourselves.

There is a rapid awakening going on today, a realization that life is more than meets the eye. Many people are becoming aware of energy, and that there are invisible forces influencing our well-being. On a collective level, we are recognizing that unseen influences like relationship stress, emotional trauma, environmental pollution, and the strain of dealing with health challenges exert powerful influence on our physical health; we are also becoming more aware that love, prayer, and intention have extraordinary healing effects. This is a quantum leap from just decades ago. Yet we haven't quite understood what it is that underlies, connects, and makes possible all these phenomena: the *etheric energy* that shapes our subtle being.

Everything contained in these pages is directed toward switching on your awareness of subtle energy and then giving you an instruction manual for how to use it in your life. It can be intimidating to discover that interferences of pollution affect your cells and that parasites of various kinds may be living within your body. It can be daunting to also make dietary changes. We will begin the journey with a calm approach that has defined natural health care through the ages: peeling away the layers to restore the vital force, using nontoxic methods and minimal intervention. You will be introduced to the hidden power of foods and ingredients that may already be in your kitchen and receive help in using them to care for your life-giving force that is the essence of who you are. One gentle step at a time, you can open to your healing potential, with Mother Nature as your ally.

I wrote *Harmonic Healing* in order to share the fundamental protocols of my clinical practice. I have used the techniques in this book in the same way, year after year, to help all kinds of people with all sorts of symptoms and concerns take their first important steps to turn their health around—and then maintain the progress through a new lifestyle of eating and living with energy. (Some of the families I care for have been with me for three generations—with the oldest members continuing the Harmonic Healing lifestyle into their nineties!) While every person's journey to health is individual, these baseline practices account for the healing that occurs. They are the groundwork that everyone does when they first become a patient and the baseline practices they continue to use to maintain balance.

Sometimes it can seem like the more you know about the challenges in our environment and the obstacles to good health, the more anxious you get about it. I invite you to be hopeful: This is a tremendous time to live healthfully. There is easier access to fresh, organic, or biodynamic food than ever before, and there are more people sharing the passion for using natural substances to heal. When you start to make the changes in this book, you will discover you are not alone, and that this knowledge—cooking nurturing soups and taking healing baths—has been the foundation of health for centuries. And by acknowledging the unseen, you will discover your innate capacity for a deeper level of self-care—an attunement to how foods make you feel and an awareness of how to use them. You can start to use these tools on an ongoing basis to stay in balance and maintain vitality, rather than letting small imbalances snowball into bigger issues.

It's not to say there will never be health challenges or problems. Each of us has been given unique tendencies toward health and disease, and we all have our individual makeup and life circumstances. There are some things we cannot change or fix. In this way of healing, we do not pray for what we want; we honor what we have been given, we come to understand that sometimes what we cannot fix or change, can be a doorway into knowing ourselves better, and finding peace, joy, and self-love. This can be a vulnerable place to be, by allowing ourselves to feel, but more importantly it can be a valuable opportunity for growth. Know that whatever you are currently experiencing or have experienced in the past, you can be influenced by subtle energy and restoring your vital energy will create health and balance in life.

Medicine today has adopted a vocabulary of fighting: When you are sick, you are often told to battle the illness and fight back against it. If you have been suffering or uncomfortable in your body for some time, I want to pave a kinder and gentler path for you to get to the other side and begin to feel better. It starts by peeling away some of the layers interfering with and suppressing your energy. As you do this by following the Harmonic Healing program, you may find your way back to your original state—the blueprint of who you are. You can begin to know what people on earth have always known: that food heals, positive thoughts heal, love heals, water heals, and conscious breathing heals. You will also discover that subtle medicine is *peaceful* medicine. And with each choice you make, adopting a new way of eating or a new method of caring for yourself, *you* create that peace within. As any true healer will say, the healer does not heal you; the healer helps you to release the blocks interfering with your natural energy, so that you can heal yourself.

What follows are the first steps to doing this, so that the power of health is in your hands to use today, tomorrow, and for many years to come.

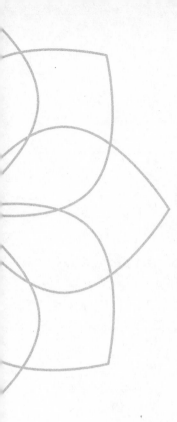

# PART ONE

# Enter the Subtle: Discovering the Unseen Aspects of Health

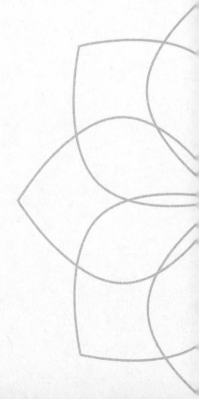

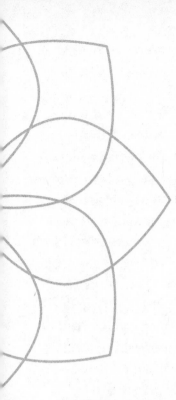

## Chapter 1

# Vitality: Your Healing Potential

There is a reservoir of energy lying just beyond the limits of your perception, and its purpose is to give you life. For millennia health and healing have been a relationship with the balance of this energy, which is a universal force that brings life to everything in existence.

This energy is known by many names across many traditions of medicine and insight. It is called *chi* in China and *ki* in Japan, *prana* in India, and etheric force or the Odic force in esoteric philosophy. Mystical Hebrew traditions refer to it as *ruach*—the breath of life. And in anthroposophical medicine, which emerged as the Western distillation of Eastern mysticism and theosophy in the early twentieth century, it is called the creative force.

I know it as *etheric energy,* an energy that exists to bring life to the body and without which the glorious physiological composition of the body would be organized and ready but not enlivened—like a brilliantly designed machine without a power cord. *Etheric* tells you something of this energy's elusive nature, for the word *ether* refers to the subtlest substance in existence, finer than light and barely perceptible by the senses. In the grandest sense, etheric energies pulsate across the vacuum of space, creating a field of creative potential that some know as consciousness, others call the zero-point field, and still others know to be the Om, the primordial sound and light.

Within you, the etheric energy is equally magnificent. It is the subtle energy that animates the physical body, fueling its cascade of functions and quietly vibrating in the empty spaces as an unseen reserve tank—the energy your body draws from to grow, reproduce, and heal. It exists within you, throughout you, and around you as a field of potential energy. Through a harmonious relationship of subtle to physical, your body transforms this potential into physical energy from the moment you are born until the time that you pass.

In homeopathy we call your body's innate ability to heal its *vital force*. Samuel Hahnemann, the father of homeopathy, referred to it as the "spirit-like" and dynamic subtle energy that drives our biological activity. From my observation and understanding of homeopathy, the vital force is what we were given as our original life force when we took our first breath, and that stays with us until we finish our journey here.

You don't have to do anything to get a vital force; you have it when you are born, it leaves with you when you die, and in between it is your body's breath of life.

You don't have to labor or exert effort to get "more" of it, for the nature of this energy is universal, omniscient, and omnipresent, and as long as you are living, it is there for you.

Yet there is a responsibility that comes with this precious gift, and that is to nourish and protect this subtle energy through the choices you make each day. When you do this, you create a state of harmony within yourself and with Mother Nature. And you create an energetic force field that radiates outward, like a protective interface or shield between your body and the taxing invisible forces from radiation, and environmental pollution.

If the words *harmony* and *coherence* remind you of music, that connection is apt. In subtle medicine, they are the energetic states that, along with a third musical term, *resonance,* help to create the inner conditions from which your vital good health, resilience against stressors and parasites, graceful aging, and recovery from unexpected injury arise. Harmony and coherence on the energetic level of the body keep your instrument in tune and your rhythms humming in sync.

## The Nature of Etheric Energy

Throughout time and across all cultures, people have understood that there are natural laws governing the workings of the universe, keeping it in balance, and coordinating its functioning. At the cosmic level, invisible forces keep the planets rotating and orbiting; electromagnetic forces allow our earth to have a field conducive to life—while gravity keeps us grounded here! At the personal level, unseen forces keep our bodies in balance and help coordinate our functions; the primary of these is the etheric energy, the invisible *impetus* for life.

The world's many schools of natural medicine—from India's Ayurveda to China's traditional medicine and Tibetan medicine to Native American healing, homeopathy, sound and distance healing, and more—have distinctive ways of naming and describing this energy. They have different practices for accessing, balancing, and stimulating it as needed, from physical practices like qigong and *pranayama* to therapeutic modalities using hands, needles, herbs, or energetic distillations to prayer and nature-based ceremony. Yet they are united around three similar understandings of its nature.

> The etheric energy within us is the etheric energy of the whole cosmos. It is the universal life force that flows through all of nature, from flora and fauna to soil, air, water, minerals, crystals, and Mother Earth herself. It is this unifying field that helps us feel connected and not separate.
>
> Etheric energy is the origin of health; and disease results when this energy becomes suppressed, blocked, or incoherent.
>
> The etheric field connects our body, emotional experience, mental processes, and spiritual reality, and is the

gateway to our higher nature. As the connector, it is the essence of a holistic approach to health.

Most of us can't see the body's subtle energy, or hear, touch, taste, or smell it. But we can detect it with a finer sense of feeling. It's what we might feel at the end of stretching and expanding our body in a yoga practice, savoring an expansive state in which body, mind, and emotions feel peacefully integrated—no one dominating more than the others, all resonating as one.

It's what buoys our body and lifts our spirits when we step into the great outdoors after too long inside, because the subtle energy of Mother Earth grounds our body and balances our energy.

You may have experienced this energy if you have ever received a healing massage or acupuncture treatment and felt yourself relaxing deeply into a space of restoration and repair, or if you have taken a homeopathic remedy like arnica after an injury and mitigated the expected pain, bruising, and swelling—benefiting from the homeopathic remedy stimulating the vital force, your body's healing energy, working in you.

Or you might not feel any of those things. Perhaps, like many people, you are familiar with this energy by its *absence;* the way it feels when its normal frequency is weak. After days of traveling on planes or living in fluorescent-lit offices, you may feel drained of your normal energy and feel tired.

After being taxed by demands and pulled in many directions, you feel like there's nothing left to draw from, and signs of sickness begin to show up. In the depleted energetic state, your thinking can turn negative or your mood dip low. These are typical outcomes when the etheric energy is low.

Whether you are savoring it or longing for it, the energy that you are connecting to in those moments is the same. Your etheric energy is your reserve energy—the source that sustains you and that your body draws from to carry out all its functions. In subtle medicine vernacular, it is the unmanifest energy that gives rise to the body's manifest actions of moving, transforming, circulating, and building. This can be described through the ancient Ayurvedic framework of the five elements, which are the foundational components of all living things. The unmanifest energy is the *ether*, which is the space from which all matter arises. The ether gives rise to the elements of air, fire, water, and earth, which in varying combinations and proportions express as physical, mental, and emotional functions.

But you can also describe it in more familiar terms. Etheric energy vitalizes the body's cells, tissues, fluids, organs, and glands in their many efforts: generating and then using or storing metabolic energy from oxygen and food, communicating via the electrical activity of the neurons and the chemical signaling of hormones, maintaining homeostasis (the balance of bodily systems) in innumerable ways every second, and meeting higher-intensity needs like healing, reproduction, and growth. Etheric energy is where regeneration begins, supporting your immune system to kick in when faced with a pathogen or your clotting agents to work when there is a cut. It is the catalyst of transformation—it turns a caterpillar into a butterfly—and the spark of rejuvenation, which determines how you age and evolve from one life stage to the next. The clue to its nature is in the word *vitality,* which by definition means *the power to live or grow.* This vital etheric energy is the prephysical energy that activates your body's potential: When your etheric body (see Your Subtle Bodies on page 24) is nourished and balanced, your body can do its magnificent work of creating the best possible conditions for health; when it is suppressed or taxed, your ability to defend and detoxify yourself and repair and regenerate yourself, plummets. The vital force we were given at birth is sustained by our "etheric energy," the doorway to health.

The reach and range of this unseen force includes your physical body but extends beyond the physical into your fields of thinking and emotion. Think of it as the invisible wave carrying all of what you are—the substructure from which the material body is formed, the activity of thoughts and pulses of feelings. Because it is the activating force for the body to be well, this force also has a very important quality that connects the physical to the emotional, mental, and spiritual: It is the force of your will to be, to heal, to live better, and to know more of who you are.

When I teach workshops on subtle medicine, we envision our etheric energy to be a river that moves around the body. We know that energy healers use tools like acupuncture needles, reiki, tai chi, or even visualizations to encourage that flow to keep moving, especially if they detect that the flow has become stagnant or slow. Typically we speak of this energy circulating through the body along invisible pathways—known as meridians in Chinese medicine and *nadis* in Ayurveda. This is true, yet one can *also* experience the subtle energy from one step subtler still, as a very fine electromagnetic energy that is interpenetrated with every part of the body, existing in every atom, cell, tissue, organ, and gland. At its essence, it is a *field of etheric energy* that exists in every part of you and radiates beyond your physical edges. Much like waves of light that are propagated in the vacuum of the cosmos, the ether exists in the empty space of our body.

Seen through my Eastern-trained eyes, this space of potential is the ether, the element of emptiness that all the other elements fill. Seen through a physicist's eyes, it is the subatomic space, the fabric in which electrons dance. The words to describe it do not really matter; but the awareness that there is subtle energy radiating through, in, and around us does. Though it is true that its balanced flow is key to having health, what few realize is that *flow* describes not a linear movement from point A to point B in the body but the *vibratory rate* of the energy itself.

## Evaluating the Vital Force: The Vibration of You

Almost four decades of working with women, men, and children of all ages has taught me a simple truth. Our vitality and healing potential comes from electromagnetic energy at the cellular level. In evaluating a patient, it is important to also evaluate their energy field. I want to know if the etheric energy is strong or weak and whether the body is utilizing this subtle energy. This is a very pragmatic and preventive approach to energy medicine—and not nearly as esoteric as some might expect! Your body is a vehicle that requires care on the physical level *and* subtle energetic level. This evaluation is a little like running a diagnostic test on your car. It lets me look into the unseen to measure basic functioning, and see where the blocks may be that are causing the body to struggle. To do this evaluation, I go right to the source of the healing potential and check the electromagnetic frequency of the cells.

If you could suddenly see your cells through subtle eyes, you would discover something fascinating. They have a physical makeup of chemical components that can be studied with a microscope, and they have a subtle energetic makeup that is an invisible double to the physical. At the chemical level, the cells have walls, mitochondria, and a nucleus of proteins and DNA that help them make fuel, communicate, grow, and reproduce. At the subtle level, the composition is purely energetic. Your cells are like little batteries or magnetic resonators with two poles, one electric and one magnetic, and these generate an oscillation of electromagnetic energy that is your body's creative force and is held in reserve in your etheric body (see Your Subtle Bodies, p. 24). Your physical body uses the etheric energy to run, just as a car uses its battery.

We are electric and magnetic beings at our very essence. The relationship between these opposites is a reflection of the balance and reconciliation that happens at every level of life. In much the same way that sages have described the creative force of the universe being born from the polarity of yin and yang—or in yogic terms, the primordial Om born of Shakti and Shiva—our essential life force arises from the pulsation of electricity and magnetism across a field of space.

When I measure etheric energy, it is the frequency emanating from the patient's cells—a little like a metal detector picking up the frequency of gold or silver!—and then evaluate the frequencies of the interferences that exist at the prephysical level. One of my tools in this endeavor is a ferromagnetic pendulum, a simple device that has a long lineage in energy medicine. In a similar manner to a reiki master tuning in to the qualities of the energy field through their hands or an Ayurvedic doctor taking the subtle pulses in the wrist, it allows me to contact the etheric field of the body, and is scientific and analytical—a testament to the brilliance of my mentor Dr. Parcells.

In radiesthesia, we measure the etheric energy field through a blood spot from the patient's finger. As long as the patient has a life force, the crystalline structure of the minerals in their dry blood spot will emanate an electromagnetic field. Like tuning in to signals of a quartz crystal in a radio, we can tune in to this field and measure the etheric body of the person. Furthermore, the life force can be measured remotely, from anywhere on the planet. It is because the earth has an electromagnetic field and we are one in this field of the earth.

When used in this system of analysis, the pendulum picks up the electrical polarity of the cells and resonates accordingly, giving me visual and kinesthetic information about the electromagnetic flow. The results of evaluation are scientific: Trained practitioners evaluating the same field will get the same measurement, because their pendulum is simply picking up the vibrational frequency of the energy field within a closed circuit, without any subjective interpretation of the results involved.

Think of it instinctually. Electricity is the fast-moving charge of action that we need to live, but electricity in excess can have aggravating, overheating, and inflammatory qualities. Magnetism is the slow-moving force that attracts and repels other forces, allowing our body to take in what it needs and get rid of what it doesn't so that homeostasis can be maintained. Too much magnetism can have heavy, turgid, and oppressive qualities—an antilife effect.

Just as all of nature seeks balance in order to perpetuate and regenerate, so does the etheric energy in your cells. If the electric charge of the cells is too strong or the magnetic pull dominates, the frequency of this fine energy gets disrupted and distorted; the etheric energy cannot radiate coherently and its force field around the body—similar to what you may know as *wei qi* or protective energy—is weak. It is as if the circuit is disturbed and the light that should shine brightly is glitchy or dim. Conversely, when the electricity and magnetism oscillate in a peaceful way, the energy radiates in organized, coherent patterns, creating a strong energetic field. Because the subtle nature of our body directly influences its physical nature, this energetic state translates into a level of integrity, resiliency, and liveliness in the cells that—to put it very simply—keeps you feeling and functioning at your best!

What determines the peaceful conditions for this play of life-sustaining energy? A nourished and balanced state in the cells, which comes predominantly from the electromagnetic potential of the food you eat, the air you breathe, and the water you drink, and from the types of thoughts you think and the feelings you feel.

### VISUALIZING SUBTLE ENERGY

Visualizing and evaluating etheric energy emanations have been revealed in many ways: Rudolf Steiner, the founder of anthroposophical medicine, taught medical doctors a technique of defocusing the eyes in order to perceive the etheric field of energy around the body; an early modern technology called Kirlian photography captured images of the etheric energy of plants and humans, and today cutting-edge scientists are observing and measuring biophotons, weak pulsations of energy and information from the cells. In Dr. Parcells's medical radiesthesia system of analysis, the kinesthetic reaction in a closed field with the use of pendulum is another way to see the etheric energy.

## The Resonance Effect

When an energy evaluation reveals a coherent pattern, I know my patient is following the guidelines he or she has been given. Making lifestyle changes, doing therapeutic baths, following the dietary recommendations and sourcing food grown in uncontaminated rich healthy soil. Plants that are grown in this way, *organically*, have higher levels of minerals creating a strong etheric energy field that will nourish us. Although sunlight, exercise, fresh water, and clean air are necessary to our vital force, it is our food that is our *primary* source of etheric energy.

When fresh, clean organic food replete with etheric energy enters our system, its electromagnetic frequency supports and strengthens our frequency due to *resonance:* the law that similar frequencies of energy amplify each other when they come into contact.

Likely you know resonance as a feeling within yourself. We often say that a person, place, or idea "resonates" with us, and even if we aren't quite sure what it means, we know how it feels: It feels good and right to be in a relationship with that person, place, or idea. I see this as a harmony of two energy systems interacting, with the new stimulus adding a beneficial or amplifying effect to the existing one. In music, a resonant vibration of a note amplifies and strengthens the sound of a similar note. If a violin string tuned to the note of C is played, its vibrating sound waves vibrate the C strings of any other nearby instruments, and as a result of this harmony, the note gets stronger. In you, the electromagnetic field of the cells in the medium of the water in your body creates a unique resonance; this combination of physical and subtle factors creates a system that is constantly in relationship with other frequencies, harmonizing with resonant ones and tolerating, or struggling with, non-resonant ones. It is like a radio receiver that picks up clear music in one moment and jarring static in another.

In its simplest expression, Harmonic Healing is about creating sympathetic resonance in your inner environment so that your cells exist in coherence, balance, and harmony. As medicines through the ages have known, the best way to do this is through close contact with nature.

## Mother Earth: Our Great Provider

The frequencies of our cells have an affinity with the frequencies of the natural world. Starting more than six thousand years ago, the ancient sciences of Ayurveda and Chinese medicine taught that we are not separate from our environment; we exist in an interdependent and cooperative relationship with it. The understanding that we are a microcosm of the macrocosm centers on our shared energetic nature, because the field of life-sustaining energy that pervades the entire cosmos is what translates to life-giving energy in our bodies. While we have the capacity to absorb frequencies of etheric energy directly from the cosmos—a capacity that gets developed the more we purify our systems and connect to our higher nature, as the yogis taught—the nourishing energy of vitality primarily comes through the channels of the earth.

The deeper understanding of earth's subtle energy gets quite esoteric—I see it as a three-part relationship of the forces of electricity, magnetism, and gravity—but the key idea is that earth's electromagnetic field is a mediator that transforms the cosmically generated, "of the ethers" energy into a form your cells can resonate with. This is why traditional medicines teach that a lifestyle of clean food, good water, and pure air, as well as honoring nature in acts of gratitude, is the bedrock for health— and why drinking from a mountain spring, eating berries plucked from wild vines, and spending time with your feet on the earth or in the ocean makes you feel as if your batteries are getting recharged. The balanced and peaceful frequencies of these things resonate with your cells, amplifying and strengthening your etheric field, which in turn funds and supports your body's extraordinary network of self-regulating systems to stay well. You then, in turn, create a strong field around you, helping to amplify and strengthen the energy of the collective earth field!

Through the ages, health care has been based on simple practices: tending to the digestive fire so that the food transfers its subtle energy to your cells, practicing conscious breathing exercises to access more of the energy from the air, and using movement of the body (like asanas, tai chi, and qigong) to either stimulate or calm the subtle energy in the body. When outside intervention is required, it has traditionally been rooted in the use of plant medicines, minerals, herbs, tonics, tinctures, oils, and essences. These medicines reflect that it is the combination of the chemical compounds and the etheric energy of these substances that resonates with your field and stimulates your vital force to heal.

You could do a deep dive into traditional systems of medicine to know yourself more deeply, or you could follow simple protocols to maintain peace within: Eat wholesome foods from the healthiest environment possible, without chemicals and additives; spend time outdoors when you can and honor—or simply enjoy!—the ground beneath your feet; and make the best choices in food and lifestyle available to you, to help Nature maintain her original, unpolluted, and energetically balanced state. And tend to yourself kindly, with some healthy reverence and self-love! The relationship we have with nature has a great deal of mystery to it, and for some of us it is one of the most profound relationships in our lives. Yet it is oriented around a very simple truth. Just like every living thing in your environment, including Mother Earth, you are both physical and subtle; chemical and electromagnetic. You are what you see, and you are what you don't see, and health comes when your attention falls equally on both.

## YOU ARE ONE, MADE OF FIVE

Many of the ancient health sciences are oriented toward detecting and resolving the imbalances in the forces that carry the vital energy into, through, and around the body. In the Vedic tradition of India, which has shaped my worldview, these are known as the five elements: the earth of our structure, the water of our emotions, the fire of our digestion, the air of our thoughts, and the ether, our supersubtle vital force! The elements are a framework for understanding the changing dynamic of health at every moment, and you will get glimpses of them throughout this book, for they can help you connect to shifts in your body's and mind's natural state of balance. The combinations of air, fire, and water in the human body are referred to as the *doshas*. They are the three elemental forces, known as *vata*, *pitta*, and *kapha*, through which the intelligence of the body works and performs its functions. These are what affect the changing dynamic of how you feel and function and are what practitioners typically attend to when evaluating health. Ether, along with food from the earth, balances the energy of the three doshas. This understanding (*tridosha*) shapes the use of food as medicine and my reverence for healing plants, for they, just like us, are the glorious combination of ether plus earth.

Your personal field of etheric energy is not just the animating force of your body; it is your individual connection to the collective etheric field that has long been probed, explored, and described through both science and sacred practice. Some call this the quantum field; others call it consciousness. It has been seen as the field of love that holds the created and uncreated realms or the gravitational field that holds the information of our creation. There is a shared understanding that there is a unified energetic field that holds and transmits not just the energy of life but all the information of life as well, and in which every part influences the rest.

The etheric field is your source of life energy and the field in which healing happens. When you connect to it, you gain access to unlimited potential. With hands, intention, or prayer, a healer can connect to the one field and direct energy to your body to heal through the etheric field. Because it supersedes three-dimensional concepts of time and space, it also can be accessed for distance healing. Now imagine the power that opens to you when you discover your subtle nature: Through your hands, your thoughts, your intention, and your prayers, you can connect to the power to give and receive healing to yourself and to others, if you have their permission to do so.

When I see a coherent energy pattern, I know a few more things about the patient beyond diet. She is probably taking some measures to avoid toxic exposures and supporting her body's detoxification systems. She may even have been actively practicing methods to counter stress, and she likely has opportunities to connect positively with others, for the energetic frequencies of peacefulness and love also create sympathetic resonance in the subtle fields, helping to nourish the vital force and thereby stimulating the healing potential. This patient would likely be feeling quite well. But she is the outlier today—I wouldn't expect to see this kind of evaluation until after a few weeks on her Liver-Cleansing Program. Because much more typically, the first evaluation reveals imbalances in the electromagnetic field of the cells—an immediate clue that she, like almost everybody today, is experiencing the effects of the first block to the etheric field: pollution.

## Your Subtle Bodies: The Origin of a Holistic Approach

Just as your cells have a physical reality and a subtle reality, so does your whole body. The aspect of your body that is a conduit for and transmitter of subtle life-giving energies is called the etheric body. The physical and etheric bodies are not two separate entities; they have been called the physical/etheric double, or physical and etheric blueprint, as they are two aspects of the body as one and coexist naturally in a double helix. Any consideration of energy medicine involves acknowledging both.

The etheric body is interpenetrated with your physical body like a sheer sheath or fabric made of very subtle threads of light. These threads or circulatory pathways are the *nadis* and meridians and create an intricate crisscrossing web of energy.

The etheric body is not visible to the eye, unless you develop the skills of supersubtle perception, which may allow you to detect it as a field of light around the physical form; this is why the etheric body is also sometimes called the light body. Consider it the unseen mirror or double of the physical. It is as much a part of you as your muscles and tissues, and it is the most important instrument you possess, because it is where the vital energy is received, assimilated, and transmitted to the physical through the gateways known as chakras: wheels or centers of energy located at the seven major endocrine glands of the body. The chakra-endocrine center is the portal through which life-giving subtle energy and invisible forces from the environment activate the body in supportive or stressful ways, and as such they are an important area of attention in Harmonic Healing (see box on p. 27).

The etheric body also holds the information or blueprint for all the body's functioning in an invisible template of growth and regeneration. I have found that the majority of diseases that manifest physically originate, unseen and unacknowledged, in the etheric body. Furthermore, it is the way into a deeper experience of yourself. Just as a well-made coat has "facing" material between the visible outer cloth and the unseen inner lining, the etheric body is the connecting field between your physical body and your invisible fields of thinking and feeling. The etheric energy moves through all these layers, connecting them in communication, allowing thoughts to move peacefully and emotions to be felt, processed, and released. This inherent connection is why, when your etheric body is in balance, your mental and emotional states feel calm, clear, and collected, and when it is depleted, the experience can easily turn negative.

What may surprise you is that you can evaluate both aspects of yourself using energy evaluation. Physical matter is at its essence energy; the physical or manifest energy is simply vibrating at a more condensed, or denser and slower, rate than the quick-moving and unmanifest etheric. Thus your physical and etheric bodies vibrate at their own relative frequencies, which can be detected with low-tech evaluation tools that detect vibration, such as the pendulum and determination board that Dr. Parcells mastered and taught. When we are vibrating at an optimal rate, it means the physical-etheric body is coordinated: The etheric energy is vitalizing the physical form, and it feels good to be in your body! This coordination can then influence the other subtle fields. A state of harmony in the physical-etheric body creates a ripple effect that spreads through the rest of you, resonating from one field to the next. I see it as the fields becoming more coordinated.

What you might experience is feeling more in touch with the different parts of yourself, and more space, and more peace.

In yogic philosophy, these subtle fields of etheric, emotional, and mental energies are known as the subtle bodies, or *koshas*. They are sheaths of energy that expand outward from the physical body in a continuum, constantly communicating with one another, affecting one another in a simultaneous and nonlinear way and ultimately connecting you to your higher soul purpose and expression. These organized bodies of energies are at the original root of our understanding of our holistic nature—it's where the phrase "mind, body, spirit" came from and is the very foundation of my knowledge of the multidimensional nature of health.

The mental body, which governs how we think, and the emotional body, which governs how we feel, get attention when you are approaching wellness multidimensionally. They are just as important as the physical and chemical constituents of blood, flesh, and bone. With the use of homeopathic remedies, imbalances in these fields can be addressed to encourage shifts at the physical-etheric, emotional, and mental level. I always *start* by attending to the balance of the electromagnetic energy and the balance of the physical-etheric energy, by attending to the very basic elements of life—the food you eat, the water you drink, the air you breathe (and the way you breathe it)—through nutritional modifications, cleansing of environmental pollution, and lifestyle shifts in order to initiate this greater state of coordination and inner harmony from the inside out.

When we recognize the etheric force field, we gain entry into a multidimensional approach to health and recognize how interconnected the physical and nonphysical aspects of ourselves truly are. Through this paradigm, we begin to understand how stress at the level of the subtle can affect us physically, mentally, and emotionally at once. Following a protocol for restoring balance at the level of energy, such as the program you will find in

Part Two, offers relief from a health-care paradigm built around compartmentalization. It treats the whole self, rather than serving the needs of the body with one set of tools (and typically one kind of doctor), the state of mind with another set, and the emotional condition with another still.

## THE ENDOCRINE SYSTEM: THE SPARK PLUGS OF LIFE

The seven chakras are wheels of subtle energy that are the connections between the etheric and the physical. Each chakra (etheric) corresponds to an endocrine gland (physical), whereby energy moves through the body. Specifically, crown chakra/pineal gland, ajna (third eye) chakra/pituitary gland, throat chakra/thyroid gland, heart chakra/ thymus gland, solar plexus chakra/pancreas, sacral chakra/gonads, and base chakra/adrenal glands. These endocrine glands secrete hormones that communicate throughout the body to regulate many of its functions. These include the processes of growing and developing; maintaining homeostasis (or body balance) through temperature, fluid balance, heart rate, and blood pressure; metabolizing food into energy and regulating hunger and weight; and initiating responses to external stimuli. They also include the processes of reproduction and the regulation of the sleep cycles we depend on for restoration, healing, immune response, and weight management to occur. Think of the endocrine glands as the spark plugs of the body, activating and vitalizing all the processes of life.

Seen through a harmonized point of view—in which subtle and physical are two aspects of one—the chakras and the endocrine glands are like the keyholes that open the doors to vitality. As such, they receive considerable attention in Harmonic Healing. They sit together as centers where vital etheric energy is received and absorbed into the etheric body and distribution points from which the vital force emanates around the body, sparking and supporting its physical needs. As you will discover, this gives them a special status—and a special vulnerability! Frequencies of all kinds, including stressful ones, exert a strong effect on the endocrine glands—as you'll discover in the next chapter, the adrenals take a particularly direct hit—and in an energy medicine evaluation, I often observe that the chakras are out of balance as a result. The next step is not to try to fix any imbalance that presents itself or to change the way the chakras pulsate or spin! Rather, this information is used as an indicator to look more deeply at that area of the body in a multidimensional way; the cause of the chakra imbalance may be an interference or block at the physical, etheric, mental, or emotional level. This is where the story of healing becomes highly individualized—and uniquely interesting.

In the first level of Harmonic Healing, and in the effort to restore vitality and overall well-being, our focus falls primarily on two chakras or energy centers of the body: the base chakra, which is the seat of the adrenal glands and the locus where environmental stress makes its first impact, and the solar plexus chakra, the seat of digestion and detoxification and the area where subtle energy from food is absorbed and processed. You will learn more about these in the chapters to come.

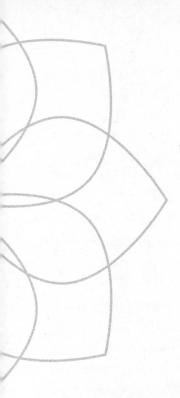

Chapter 2

# Identifying Interferences: The Invisible Forces That Affect Health

hree patients arrive at my office from different walks of life. The first is a finance executive who frequently travels by plane, faces high loads of daily stress, and finds herself overly fatigued and often sick with sinus infections. The second is a single father who has been struggling with the symptoms of Lyme disease for some time, see-sawing between feeling a little better and a lot worse, never able to find equilibrium. The third is a young teacher just starting her career in the big city, challenged by digestive issues that have her constipated on some days and hit by diarrhea on others. Her dietary changes have helped make some headway but have not resolved the issues, and managing this chronic condition is sapping her energy and, more important, her will.

I observe each person as they settle in for their consultation. Before a word is exchanged, their physical appearance transmits information about their vitality and guides me to places in their system where there is weakness that may be creating disharmony. If the pupils of their eyes are dilated, it can indicate that the adrenals are exhausted and stress levels are high, or it can indicate the presence of shock in the subtle fields. If the hair is thin, very likely the digestion or thyroid is out of balance or the kidneys may be overworking. If the skin is irritated or flush with rashes, it's a sign that there could be distress in the liver, intestines, or lungs.

When one practices energy medicine, the first glance at the patient is also a subtle look. For example, shock can be seen as dullness or a grayness in the energy field, as it is a disruption in the communication between the etheric and the physical body. When the etheric body has vitality, it radiates through the network of subtle pathways, illuminating the body with a bright radiance, not a dull gray field.

The executive, the father, and the teacher may not share all the same symptoms, but each one presents the same gray haze. This does not elicit alarm; it is simply a piece of information that brings awareness to something normally in the shadows. It signals that they, like all of us, are living in a sea of interferences that are invisibly disrupting the healing potential, negatively affecting their endocrine system or "spark plugs" of vitality and burdening their organs of detoxification. These patients simply haven't yet become aware of how these interferences, which include pollution, stress, and shock, affect their subtle bodies and have yet to learn that there are tools to neutralize them. Which is why, whether they have sought out Harmonic Healing in order to resolve generalized low immunity, low energy, or a chronic condition, we always start at the same place: the balance of the electromagnetic energy in their etheric field.

## The Sea of Environmental Pollution

Imagine a day in the average modern life: Breakfast comes out of a cardboard box, sterilized container, or plastic bag, laced with preservatives that lengthen its shelf life. Coffee is spiked with an exotic flavor that nature couldn't produce and is combined with a cream substitute made of chemicals and sugar. At lunch and dinnertime, the ingredients on the plate bear traces of the chemicals that helped them to grow and complex enhancers derived from a lab and, oftentimes traces of the aluminum cookware used in cooking or baking too.

The day takes place overwhelmingly indoors, in buildings whose air contains gases from the man-made materials used to build and furnish it, including things we would never guess are present, such as traces of mercury emitted by the compact fluorescent lightbulb illuminating our workstation or by the radiation from the laptop on which we type. Outside, heavy metals from manufacturing and energy production pervade the atmosphere and invisibly contaminate the air that we breathe and the food that we eat.

When we get ready for the day, we might apply an array of products to our skin, nails, and hair that contain petroleum-derived chemicals like phthalates and parabens, which can get absorbed into our bodies. And when we dress, our clothing may comprise fibers sprayed with contaminants or plastics that can transmit their chemicals into the body. Or it may have been laundered with synthetic fragrances that smell appealing but subtly disturb our hormones.

Throughout the day, at home, at work, at school, and even in transit, webs of Wi-Fi transmit wireless radiation in pulsing frequencies; and the devices, the home systems, and the infrastructure on which they run keep reverberating around us all through the night.

For some there may even be a plane trip thrown into the mix—a source of gamma-ray radiation, due to the proximity to the sun. Into this disruptive mix a ceaseless river of personal and professional demands presents itself to us daily, requiring constant energy and attention while depriving us of the rest and recovery time we need. And this drama is unfolding on a uniquely vulnerable stage: a modern-day body that typically has a weakened vital force, due in part to the depleted electromagnetic potential of so much of our food. Individually, these disturbances could be aggravating to our health; taken together, they add up to a continuum of ever-increasing interferences that no one in even the very recent past could have envisioned.

I categorize these disturbing factors collectively as "pollution." Just as pollution puts undue stress on the earth, influencing ecosystems and affecting climate change, pollution in the human system interferes with our cells' frequencies while depleting our organs and glands. Pollution—just like healing!—is multidimensional: The stressors include heavy metals and chemicals in our food, our water, and our air; radiation in our space; and disturbances in our personal relationships and our thoughts.

All these things have an energetic dimension and a physical dimension. To be well in this milieu of unseen forces requires looking at both the physical and the etheric energetic aspects of our bodies and the environment in which we live.

Physicians and healers, regardless of specialty, share the same concerns about the surge in collective ill health and suffering and together are shedding light onto what was for years an unacknowledged subject. Decades after I began detecting heavy metals and chemicals through the practice of radiesthesia, their impact continues to intensify as we embrace more and more technology in our daily lives and also because our etheric fields are weakened from the interference of environmental pollution on our electromagnetic energy.

Interference creates the opposite of resonance: Instead of amplifying and supporting the energy pattern of the body, the disturbance makes it incoherent—the radio receiver is broadcasting static, not songs, and the sound is scrambled. In this environment, the little batteries of the cells lose their power; the reserve energy of the body becomes weak, and the etheric field loses its energy. The endocrine glands and the liver and gallbladder, meanwhile, work overtime trying to keep the worst effects of the pollutants at bay as the digestive fire struggles to derive the necessary nutrients from food, while our immune system weakens. It's no surprise that the vehicle of our physical body begins to suffer—with the batteries losing charge, the spark plugs overworked and exhausted, the safety features degraded, and the engine and oil lines clogged, how could it not?

## The Three Laws of Frequency

We are more aware than ever before about the challenges of chemicals, heavy metals, and radiation. You may know a little about the very long life span of unwanted metals such as aluminum, lead, and mercury in the body, and that they accumulate in our tissues and bones to deleterious effect; if you follow the topic closely, you may even have read how some of the chemicals in our environment work synergistically with metals, helping to transport them through the gut wall and into the bloodstream. Chances are that you already make daily choices to reduce the impact of environmental pollution where you can. You might limit seafood to reduce exposure to mercury and waterborne chemicals and audit personal-care products to avoid petrochemicals absorbing through the skin. Perhaps you avoid sodas with fake sweeteners like aspartame or try to use a headset with a cell phone or its speaker function whenever possible. These choices are good ones, yet for most of us there is still a missing link about *why* we are making them. Why do stressors that are invisible to the eye, or that are only present in very small or even imperceptible amounts, have such an effect? To understand the *full* disruptive potential of these invisible forces, step beyond the materialist mind-set and discover three laws of frequency.

## The First Law: Frequency Affects Frequency

Everything that exists has a frequency. Be it a physical substance in solid, liquid, or gas form (like a noxious chemical in your cleaning products) or a nonphysical radio wave coming from your Wi-Fi router (or even a thought or emotion), *everything* is at its essence frequency, vibrating at different densities—the slower the vibration, the more solid and condensed the matter. Some frequencies resonate and create harmony in our body; others interfere and create disharmony.

We use the laws of energy to a healing effect in homeopathy, one of the subtlest medicines that is available to an energy medicine practitioner and now widely available over the counter. In homeopathy a standard procedure is employed through a sequence of distillations and vigorous shaking that energizes the physical substance of a chosen plant, mineral, or animal matter (such as sepia, the ink of the cuttlefish) until nothing but the energetic essence—its etheric energy pattern or information blueprint—is left in the water, as a frequency. This water is then used to infuse tiny sucrose-lactose pellets taken by mouth and, depending on the remedy's frequency, begins to resonate with the frequency of a patient's physical-etheric body, mental body, or emotional body, stimulating the vital force. In homeopathy it is the *vibration* of the substance that is the medicine, and the *smaller* the dose the higher the potency and the *more* potent the effect can be. If the remedy is well chosen according to homeopathy's Law of Similars, it can initiate a stimulation to the person's vital force to heal. As practitioners and patients know from experience, though energetic frequencies are invisible, their effects are very real.

This first law of frequency opens potential for healing—energy heals—and also reminds us to care for ourselves on an energetic as well as a physical level in our increasingly polluted environment. Our bodies have physical barriers like the skin, the microbiome, and secretions like mucus that protect us against unwanted impacts and invaders; they also have an unseen wall of energy protecting us—our etheric field.

## The Second Law: The Stronger Frequency Will Take Over the Weaker One

Heavy metals like aluminum, lead, mercury, cadmium, and arsenic, as well as industrial chemicals, emanate strong magnetic frequencies—these are the low, slow vibrations that pull your cellular energy down. Radiation, meanwhile, exerts overly electric frequencies—these are the high-speed, agitated vibrations that aggravate the cell energy. Each is an extreme—these are the two poles of the electromagnetic balance—and each has the potential to dominate the energy in your cells. Think of it like loud voices drowning out quieter ones at a party—the quieter ones may be speaking kinder, smarter words, but the loud ones drown them out. When evaluating a patient's etheric energy, I look for the presence of these interferences at the cellular level, because they indicate that the three main forms of pollution from the environment, heavy metals and chemicals on the one hand and radiation on the other, are present. The *degree* to which they are present will vary considerably depending on how the person eats—organic or not, made-at-home or dining out—how many interferences fill their environment, their location, and their lifestyle.

## The Third Law: Imbalance Most Often Occurs in the Etheric Before Occurring in the Physical

Health and disease can be detected in the etheric field even before they manifest physically. The presence of pollution often appears in the body's etheric field before it shows up physically in the tissues or fluids. If left to accumulate and persist, it can begin to create disharmony, subtly at first—by weakening the vital force and disturbing the way the endocrine glands interact with one another—and then more manifestly, as the body goes into overdrive to break down and expel what has begun to accumulate in the tissues. This is why attending to the prephysical level of health brings such benefit: We can detect imbalance early and endeavor to neutralize or resolve it before it causes bigger problems. This is also why trace amounts of contaminants can have such a disruptive effect on our well-being—they are creating an effect even before we can physically quantify them. As natural healers know, disharmony and disease are usually harder to turn around after they have manifested physically. This is why I prefer to use slow and steady preventive measures to counteract pollution that has accumulated as part of a whole lifestyle, rather than some of the more invasive clinical treatments, which can cause additional stress on the body. Since pollution is a continuous interference, it is wise to find solutions that we can use regularly.

## Disturbances in the Field

We are natural beings living in unnatural times, and we all live in the same sea of interferences. We can avoid some of the pollution around us, but unless we move off the grid entirely and disengage from the world at large, we will never avoid all of it; it is the background noise against which we live. While we do not want to live in fear or anxiety, it is wise to live with an awareness of the two polarities of pollution—chemicals and metals on the one end and radiation on the other.

## Interfering with Our Energy Field: Chemicals and Heavy Metals

Food, air, and water are the most persistent sources of exposure to chemicals and heavy metals. We ingest food daily, and if it is conventionally grown, with each bite come traces of the chemicals and heavy metals not only used in the growing process of plants (herbicides, fungicides, pesticides, and fertilizers, many of which contain both substances) but also from the groundwater used to water them, which may contain metals like arsenic and industrial pollutants. More chemical agents may be used during the harvesting, ripening, and manufacturing processes—chemicals with long, confusing names are added to foods and drinks for flavor, texture, and preservation. Meats and other animal proteins raised on these plants can contain many of the same pollutants; the pharmaceutical drugs used in the process of raising the meats exacerbates the effect. Fish can come from oceans and watersheds laced with heavy metals and chemicals from agricultural runoff and plastic waste. Because these interferences are not containable—air and water are mediums for pollution that have no boundaries—they affect us all, regardless of our dietary ideologies: When evaluated, meat eaters and vegetarians alike exhibit similar energy fields.

Food preparation adds further interference. An unacknowledged source of heavy metals in the body is the aluminum that migrates into our bodies from cookware and foils—aluminum cookware is a staple of most restaurants and many homes. This gets absorbed into the food during the cooking process without our knowing. It shows up at elevated levels in the evaluations of patients who dine out frequently—that muffin, pizza, or sauté pan used behind the scenes is almost always made of aluminum. The plastics used to wrap, store, and reheat foods are similarly problematic, as are chemicals from coated "nonstick" pans; these chemicals interfere with our hormones, the messengers of the body from the endocrine glands.

It doesn't end there. We unknowingly inhale traces of metals like lead and nanoparticles of aluminum from the air, probably the greatest source of heavy metals. Carbon monoxide from exhausts and petrochemicals from manufacturing also lace the air we breathe, especially in our cities. Sadly, many of us are starting to experience heightened exposure to these interferences when faced with natural disasters, like when smoke fills the atmosphere from wildfires, or during floods, when noxious materials lace the floodwaters. Chemical residues and traces of pharmaceutical drugs are found in the water we drink or bathe in, and we are waking up to the volume of chemicals used in intricate, and untested, combinations in products used for self-care. Medications, meanwhile, a staple of every bathroom cabinet, also fit this category—their energetic field is low and slow. Dental amalgams, a staple of dentistry in previous decades, contain up to 50 percent mercury, which has been found to leach into the tissues and become an insidious source of mercury exposure for many people. (If mercury fillings are still in your mouth, consider asking your dentist about replacing them with a less toxic choice; if your dentist recommends using them now, I suggest getting another opinion.) Heavy metals also find their way directly into the bloodstream through injection in the form of vaccines, which include nanoparticles of aluminum, often in conjunction with trace amounts of mercury—a controversial subject, but one that could also be brought out of the shadows and looked at with more clarity.

Volumes have been written on the effects of heavy metals on the body. It is known that these metals compete with the minerals in our system that our bodies need to function. Aluminum, now understood to be by far the most pervasive heavy metal in our air, is correlated with the development of Alzheimer's as well as cancer growth, and as I have observed many times, its presence helps to strengthen the powerful hold of the Lyme spirochete. Mercury has been linked to neurologic impairment, immune and digestive disorders, heart disease, metabolic syndrome, and more—mercury is considered the most dangerous metal, as it blocks hormones from their normal function in the body. Volatile organic compounds from paint and furnishings irritate the respiratory tract, and parabens from plastics can disrupt the endocrine system. Glyphosate, the active ingredient in Round Up, is the world's most widely used herbicide and has been linked to cancer, gut flora imbalance (also known as dysbiosis), and neurological impairments and is now described as a carrier for metals, helping to escort them more effectively into the body, where they can accumulate in the brain, kidneys, or bones. And heavy metals and chemicals are widely understood to be a factor in causing autism in children; I have witnessed time and again how neutralizing these pollutants has changed the cellular function. My observation has been that when pollution is addressed, the pain of fibromyalgia, Lyme disease, brain dullness, and memory issues begins to improve remarkably.

## THE INVISIBLE AMPLIFIER

The pervasive use of glyphosate in our food supply and on our gardens and public spaces is one of the most troubling influences in our environment. Glyphosate is a powerful metal binder that binds with mercury and aluminum, making them more toxic. It not only disturbs the detoxification process of the liver but also helps the metals make their way through the gut barrier and into the bloodstream. It also helps carry metals like aluminum into the brain. It is impossible to avoid glyphosate entirely, as traces of it can migrate from fields treated with chemicals into waterways and even onto organic fields. Glyphosate is also used to treat many grain and legume crops after harvesting. Choosing organic, non-GMO food is the best way of reducing the burden and protecting ourselves from this challenging herbicide.

In clinical practice I frequently detect the presence of specific pollutants that correlate clearly with a patient's line of work; a florist who handles chemically saturated floral foam blocks may have high levels of formaldehyde; a jeweler who works with antique materials can have high levels of lead, and a farmer, not surprisingly, may exhibit high levels of arsenic from spraying the apple orchard. Sometimes the pollutants are connected to lifestyle choices, like the woman who is so afraid of bugs that she overuses bug repellents in her home, or the runner who runs on the side of the road, inhaling not only the exhaust of vehicles but also the weed killers that have been sprayed on the verges. Even the golfer who plays a round in the early morning, when the dew is evaporating on the recently sprayed green, can have high levels of chemical fertilizer and weed killers.

We can work on lowering especially high levels of individual interferences as they present using detoxifying baths as a foundation—as you will learn, apple cider vinegar is our tool for neutralizing carbon monoxide. In energy medicine, however, and as the general starting point to wellness, we look at the *overall* effect of the total load of pollution. The accumulation of heavy metals and chemicals can pull down our cell energy and suppress the vital force, and the organs and systems of digestion and detoxification most particularly feel the effects. The accumulated pollution can congest the lymph system, and the heavy metals can interfere with the stomach's ability to make enough digestive juices, while hindering the function of the liver. Because the liver is so intimately connected to our will, the "heavy" quality of these unseen interferences can play out as depression and/or low energy.

Becoming aware of these interferences can be disconcerting, because short of moving to a pristine environment far from industry and cut off from technology, we cannot avoid encountering them. Yet awareness also brings great benefit; when we are able to neutralize the effects of heavy metals and chemicals, a lot of the deep health struggles we may have been engaged in become significantly easier to resolve, because these interferences have such a powerfully determining effect on whether we are well or ill. It is empowering to discover how fresh, clean, nourishing foods imbued with etheric energy support our own etheric energy field and baths can neutralize the onslaught of chemicals, heavy metals, and radiation.

When Jon came into Light Harmonics clinic, he was on the cusp of forty and dreading his birthday. Jon is a punk-rock filmmaker who doesn't follow convention, yet he felt the clichés of middle age approaching; he was getting older, slower, and heavier. This wasn't surprising, because his evaluation revealed that his levels of aluminum and other metals, as well as chemicals, were high. When asked to describe his diet, he sheepishly described Jack in the Box for breakfast and leftover Chinese food for dinner and admitted that he and fresh vegetables were not exactly friends. It wasn't age that was getting to him; it was the contamination accumulating from his steady diet of takeout and frozen meals that had pulled down the energy of his cells and weakened his vitality. The puffiness in his face, bags under his eyes, and extra pounds creeping onto his body were just a few of the consequences. Unbeknownst to him, this weakened environment was causing his symptoms. To turn the downhill trajectory around, Jon's first step would be to neutralize heavy metals, chemicals, and radiation with regular detoxifying baths while clearing out of his life the most commonly ingested sources of pollution—the processed and packaged foods he had come to rely on while immersed in making his films. As his vitality returned, so did his enthusiasm to take good care of himself, and he even became passionate about sourcing fresh and local food.

## Aggravating and Disturbing Your Energy Field: Radiation

The definition of the word *radiation* is energy that is transmitted from a source, moves through space, and is absorbed by something else. Natural radiation is always present on earth, thanks to the electromagnetic fields of free electrons dancing on the surface and lightning bolts that charge the field.

The spectrum of *man-made* electromagnetic radiation includes a range of wavelengths of energy that are much stronger than nature's and far more complex; it includes extremely low-frequency magnetic fields that are generated wherever electricity flows and emanates from power boxes, power lines, and the wiring in our homes—if we live too close to power sources or have faulty wiring in our walls, the fields can be strong enough to disturb the frequency of our cells. It also includes the high-frequency radio waves of wireless technology; these are especially complex and layered in their impact, for they are pulsing with the electricity of the power source, the frequencies of the wavelengths, jarring signal characteristics, and data that is being carried on the waves. Today we are almost never out of range: High-frequency radio waves and ultra-high-frequency microwaves from cell phones, cell antennae and towers, computers and routers, Bluetooth devices, and, increasingly, home appliances like televisions, refrigerators, home security systems, and baby monitors are by their very nature energetically and biologically disruptive. Our minds might overlook the inconvenient truth, but our energy bodies do not.

In the years since starting to practice energy analysis, I have seen the interference from radiation grow and grow. It correlates with the explosion of wireless radiation into every nook and cranny of our empty space—our collective ether field. The pervasiveness of this interference increases exponentially by the year: Homes are hooked up to systems that can run every domestic appliance through technology. Our personal Wi-Fi networks are surrounded by countless others in neighboring homes and workplaces, amplifying the impact; and smart meters installed on buildings constantly transmit utility readings to energy providers via high-intensity microwaves that affect those living and working inside. With a new era upon us as 5G wireless networks based on military-grade technology increase the burden through even more intense and disturbing frequencies, the impact of wireless radiation will be exponentially higher—and the ability to avoid it, even in seemingly quiet and peaceful areas, will get diminished.

All these exposures to radiation aggravate the electromagnetic balance of the cells. Where the interference from heavy metals and chemicals *slows and congests,* the interference from radiation *disturbs and aggravates.* The endocrine glands, which are exceptionally sensitive to frequency as the gatekeepers between the etheric and physical, get disturbed, sometimes become hypo- (low) or hyper- (overly high) functioning. Red blood cells clump together, creating a higher risk for heart disease. The body's intricate communication systems—not only hormonal but also electrical and microbial—start to get scrambled, creating all manner of havoc. Oxidative stress causes free-radical damage that, among many other things, contributes to faster aging, and the cell membrane gets harder, making it more challenging for nourishment to enter and waste to be discharged. The etheric blueprint of the body gets distorted, damaging processes of regeneration and reproduction (effects on DNA, the physical expression of the etheric template, are widely understood to be one consequence of radio-wave exposure). In this bombardment of radiation, the immune system in particular is affected as the radiation affects the spleen, the master gland of the immune system. When this occurs, sicknesses can be frequent, resiliency low, and disease processes in the weak parts of our body more prone to occur.

We are exposed to unnatural levels of radiation in other ways too. Medical technologies like X-rays and CT scans expose us to intensely disturbing, and extra-high, frequencies. The tragic reality of radioactive disasters like the Fukushima nuclear reactor meltdown impacting our oceans and air adds another layer of radioactivity into our environment that we'd be wise not to ignore—*ionizing* radiation such as the highest-frequency waves on the spectrum, gamma rays, which have the capability to break molecular bonds and create ionized atoms, which are known carcinogens. Sometimes we even innocently track radioactive material indoors: Fracking infuses radioactive material from deep in the earth into wastewater, which is then used to produce asphalt. The material can come into our homes on our shoes. Underground radiation can flow under our homes from streams that emanate naturally occurring radioactive substances. If an underground stream of water passes through radioactive material such as uranium, and if that stream flows under our bedrooms, it can interfere with sleep, affect the immune system, and create illness. (Such issues can be hard to identify, but experts trained in dowsing for water can often detect the streams and then begin to find a solution.)

One of the unusual but consistent findings during an energy evaluation is that those who fly usually have ionizing radiation of natural gamma rays in their field. This can occur as a result of flying at elevations of over 35,000 feet, when we are closer to the sun. This exposure to high frequency gamma ray radiation is unnatural and difficult for our bodies. I often find that those who fly frequently have challenged immune systems, and prescribe a sea salt and baking soda bath (described in chapter 6) after an airplane flight. (Many airlines are inadvertently increasing the amount of radiation exposure by hosting Wi-Fi in flight; the intensity of the wireless radiation gets amplified by the metal of the airplane.)

## NEGATIVE THOUGHTS

The fears and frustrations that fill our minds and the angers, hates, and anxieties that radiate from the people we interact with are also radiations that aggravate the balance of our energetic field and suppress the vital force. Mental radiations can be supportive and positive; loving encounters, prayer, and meditation all resonate and amplify our subtle energy. But tides of bad news, unkind opinions, and toxic thoughts can be as disturbing to the energetic body as any other intense radiation. Exposure to these radiations weakens our subtle energy, and if they intensify they can create a state of shock, described below. Reducing these fields' negative impact involves cultivating intentional positivity within and setting boundaries on what and who surrounds you without. Because the physical-etheric, mental, and emotional fields influence one another so deeply, these measures are as important as eating your greens if you want to enjoy health.

When radiation and heavy metals are present together, the synergy can be especially troubling: I have noticed in clinical observation that when mercury has sequestered itself in the tissues of the brain, the impact of cell-phone radiation is multiplied. Setting limits on technology use, especially for our children with their developing brains, then becomes as important as starting to neutralize the interfering metal.

All of this can seem intimidatingly out of our control, but our philosophy is not to live in fear about the radiation in our everyday environment but rather to live with awareness. We acknowledge that much of the problematic technology was developed in order to help humanity evolve and grow; but the scales have tipped out of balance. So we take action, reducing exposures through lifestyle choices where we can and taking regular care to counteract exposure and balance these fields through natural methods of clearing, like detoxifying baths and foods (such as antioxidant-rich fresh vegetables and fruits and iodine-rich seaweed) that can help to neutralize radiation.

When it comes to the forces of pollution, our modern milieu does not give us a break. The interferences persist unresolved until you begin to neutralize them. As the electromagnetic balance changes at the cellular level and the extreme fields take over, the cellular integrity becomes weak. The cells can lose their electrical charge, the energetic pattern becomes incoherent, and as a result, our reserve energy weakens, hampering our ability to heal, repair, and grow. We might feel "spent" more than normal, and when a new challenge like an injury, an upsetting encounter, or a cold or flu presents itself, we are more easily sidelined by it and find it harder to recover from. Loss of electromagnetic balance in the cells is the first step in the spiral of the disease process—and a key factor in aging, because without the balanced flow of electricity in our cells, we age faster.

The vital force dynamically adapts and adjusts to many stressors. It responds to the stimuli that challenge us by prompting the body's homeostatic and healing mechanisms to kick in. But there is a limit: When the stimuli are unrelenting, this capacity gets overburdened. Imagine it like feet pressing down fresh grass consistently, never letting up—over time, it gets harder and harder for the grass to spring back up when into this already challenged environment come the added assaults of shock.

> Deirdre was maintaining good health as a busy Los Angeles hairdresser, until she moved to New York City in 2012 to launch her own hair salon. Six months after her arrival, she began to experience strange symptoms that got progressively worse: foggy brain and anxiety, insomnia by night and extreme fatigue by day. Her energy evaluation revealed extremely high levels of radiation—which perplexed her, as her lifestyle did not involve high computer and cell-phone use. But Deirdre soon discovered that she was working and living in buildings with newly installed banks of smart

meters, which perpetually transmit utility information in two-way communication to satellites via cellular microwave signals. In addition, a hub of cell-phone antennae had been installed right outside her bedroom window. We are particularly vulnerable to high-frequency radiation when we sleep, because our parasympathetic nervous system does its restoration and healing. At that time, the combination of the meters and the antennae had overwhelmed her system. She began to experience nausea, diarrhea, hair loss, exhaustion, and anemia.

Though these invisible pressures affect all of us, they go unacknowledged by many. Deirdre was the canary in the coal mine, subjected to excessive and ongoing exposure and responding not only with uncomfortable symptoms but also with a deep level of fatigue—an indication that her vital force was low and the electromagnetic balance at the cellular level was disrupted. Determined to reclaim her health, Deirdre took action. She moved to a home without smart meters or cell antennae in order to protect herself from the worst of the excess radiation, and learned ways to lower electromagnetic field (EMF) exposure in daily life. She committed to a program of baths to neutralize the accumulation of radiation and metals, and she filled her diet with organic vegetables, including lots of beets and bitter greens and high-quality grass-fed and organic meats to rebuild her blood, and seaweed to nourish her thyroid and help neutralize the radiation.

Freed from the pressure of the most intense interferences, and nourished with extra support, Deirdre's body began to recover (like the grass springing back up after being flattened for some time). Her energy normalized, and with some time and patience her health blossomed again. Though the sickness from the radiation exposure had tested Deirdre to her core, taking control of her health had given her a profound new connection to her body. Several years after rebounding from the darkest part of her journey, Deirdre continues to take the best care possible of her liver and nourish her blood, as she continues to take her regular detoxifying baths.

## Shock: The Invisible Split

All of us have had shock in our systems, yet most of us don't know it. A shock can occur in the physical-etheric body through an injury, an allergic response, or an exposure to a toxic chemical or metal or even a noxious smell (almost like anaphylactic shock); it can come from living in a state of unrelenting fight-or-flight stress, from overindulging in certain foods (hence the term *sugar shock*), from abuse of alcohol or drugs, and even through exposure to high-powered electromagnetic fields.

It can occur in the mental body, such as through financial stress and all the worries it brings, interpersonal conflict, or abusive relations and language. Shock can also occur in the emotional body through any number of upsetting or traumatic events, such as a family ordeal, a deep personal disappointment, any kind of assault, or grief from divorce, separation, loss, or death. Living in an environment that is pervaded with fear can create shock, and tragedies and disasters on a community or national scale can create more shock, even if you are not involved directly.

While interferences disturb the electromagnetic balance of the cells, shock can create a *separation* between the physical and etheric bodies that interferes with our energy flow. A shock can be sudden and acute; it can also come on through persistent distress or chronic exposure to contaminating or toxic influences. And when we experience it, a dislodging can occur between the physical and etheric bodies; no longer can the subtle energy move easily to feed into the physical from the etheric, emotional, and mental fields. Not only does this deprive us of vitality and create persistent, sometimes crushing fatigue, but it can leave us feeling disoriented and cut off from feelings and mental clarity. Sometimes we experience anger and aggression or deep-seated fear, which we struggle to reconcile, unaware that the cause was out of our control. Shock is what often accounts for grayness in our energy field.

A shock may have occurred long ago, yet it will continue to reverberate until it is resolved or processed. The disharmony it causes in the physical-etheric body is a kind of protective mechanism, the body's way of saying "stop" to experiences it can't handle. Out of sight, shock can quietly affect us by exhausting the kidneys, the seat of the emotions in the physical-etheric body, and interfere with the functioning of the adrenals, which rise to protect us when threatened. Gradually we learn to adapt to this split, getting used to the fatigue or the mental and emotional uncoordination and developing coping techniques to get us through each day. As life goes on, we experience more shocks, and the pressures on the body continue.

Today it can feel like we are living in an age of shock; tuned in to disasters on a global scale, daily recipients of tragic details we might once not have heard. After a profound trauma like 9/11 in New York City, I dispensed homeopathic remedies for shock and grief widely—homeopathy is one of the most profound methods for clearing shock, along with cranial sacral therapy, reiki, polarity therapy, and flower and gem remedies—and helped my patients to rebuild the adrenal glands, which had responded to the shock, with supportive herbs and foods.

Traditional medicines have always seen disease as the result of blocks in the physical, etheric, mental, or emotional level, for if the life force and the healing intelligence that it carries are suppressed, disharmony can take over and initiate a dis-ease process. A block can even be at the spiritual level; when something breaks our connection to our higher nature, it can leave us isolated, lost, and cut off from our will to live. In such cases the healer's role may include encouraging the patient to take up a contemplative, meditative, or spiritual practice in order to help him acknowledge the higher source within and to restore hope.

When shock is present, you could follow diets to the letter but not be able to lose weight, or do everything you're told to avoid migraines but still get headaches; you also become particularly vulnerable to the five types of parasites, which you will meet in chapter 3, for they thrive when we are in a state of vulnerability. To heal, we attend to shock and allow the body to let it go by using gentle methods of clearing it, for if it is left unresolved, the disruption it causes to the flow of our etheric energy can make getting well more difficult.

Shock is one of the first things I check for if I detect that the etheric energy or reserve energy is low; Harmonic Healing contains various treatments or remedies for shock and grief that can light the spark of hope if it has gone dim by helping the vital force begin to move from where it was suppressed.

## The Cascade of Effects

Stressors like pollution, shock, worry, and the sheer unrelenting demands of everyday life affect us all differently; some of us have higher thresholds for physical exertion, others have stronger mental fields. Yet what is universal is the effect of the cumulative burden. When our subtle energy is balanced and our etheric field is strong, we have a measure of resistance to the whole gamut of interferences we meet. But when that protective field gets tested and weakened, the energetic defense, which is our immune system, loses its capacity to defend. The weaker this gets, the more intensely our bodies respond to threats, seeking to protect us from the bombardment. Our body wants to live in peace in the environment and will do what it can to protect and preserve life.

The first line of defense is the adrenal glands; they are our survival center, for they respond to incoming challenges by activating the whole body to be on alert. The adrenal glands play a vital role in the body's "spark plugs" or endocrine system and supporting our will to be—they contribute to our sense of grounding and our desire to live on this physical plane. All our endocrine glands, which also include the ovaries and testes, thyroid, pancreas, thymus, and pituitary and pineal glands, are distribution points where the etheric energy transfers into the physical body to energize our organs and systems. It's where the body, in a sense, taps into and uses its reserves, and is the body's energy system for that reason. By design, this system works in an intricate dance of coordination, with glands communicating with one another through energy! But when stressors are unrelenting, and the endocrine glands are on over-drive or underdrive, the distribution points get stuck and snarled, making it difficult for the energy to flow.

The adrenals are the endocrine glands that sit above the kidneys, and from a subtle energy point of view, they resonate within the wheel of energy known as the base chakra; it governs our basic survival needs and our physical will for life and is connected to the entire nervous system. When the adrenals receive the stimuli of any kind of stressor, be it interference from heavy metals, chemicals, or radiation or a physical, mental, or emotional shock, they respond to the danger. A cascade of hormones is initiated throughout the body to launch the fight-or-flight response. Survival mechanisms like inflammation are switched on, and nonurgent needs like digestion, repair, regeneration, and growth are shut down. In a state of stress, the healing potential is temporarily suppressed as the activities necessary for fighting or fleeing get all the energy available.

Over time, if this pattern persists, the conditions are created for a weakened immune system, heightened inflammation, digestive dysfunction, and disruption to carbohydrate metabolism, leading to weight gain. Excessive activity either overstimulates or exhausts these hardworking glands as they rise and fall in fight-or-flight responses. As the burden of survival ripples out to other endocrine glands, the thyroid gland attempts to take over in support. But in an energetically weakened system, the thyroid eventually tires too, leading to more fatigue, weight gain, digestive distress, and immune system dysfunction; this can even lead to a medical diagnosis of a thyroid imbalance. Because it is simpler to test the thyroid through a thyroid-profile lab test than it is to test for an imbalance in the adrenal glands, we are seeing a wave of diagnoses of thyroid dysfunction and consequent rush to use thyroid medications. In truth, this tends to miss the true adrenal cause in many cases.

And in the center of this hurricane, the slowed and congested liver and digestive organs struggle to take in nourishment, as the liver tries to detoxify the heavy metals and chemicals we have ingested, inhaled, or absorbed. Accumulated pollution can also irritate the gut wall, allowing unwanted proteins from food and pollution to cross into the bloodstream, activating an immune system response. The result of these interferences can be systemic inflammation, which flares up in weak or vulnerable areas of the body depending on our individual constitution and our health history—it could be the stomach, the intestines, the joints, the prostate, the ovaries and reproductive center and sites of fertility, the skin, or other areas. Where the fire of inflammation burns, pain and distress follow.

A state of adrenal stress and exhaustion is extremely common today; yet what many do not realize is that the causes are not only mental and emotional stress. They also include the bombardment of pollution and interference to the cellular balance, and the resulting overreaction of the adrenals. Clearing the polluting interferences regularly to restore the balance of cellular energy and restore the vital force is a pivotal aspect of the Harmonic Healing lifestyle. With the detoxifying baths, we do our maintenance work to keep the daily bombardment of pollution down so that we do not reach the tipping point in which organs and systems struggle to keep up with their function or begin a downward spiral. Meanwhile, we also nourish ourselves with good food to strengthen our etheric field. I have found that the combination of these two habits, along with lifestyle changes to avoid unnecessary exposures, can allow us to enjoy our lives in this increasingly complex modern milieu—and this is even the case for those who may already be experiencing illness from elevated levels of pollution. Calmly and methodically, we can begin to bring these levels down.

There is another very important reason to do this maintenance work. It has to do with the *second* unseen factor behind fatigue, ill health, and a whole spectrum of struggles from mild to extreme. Pollution in the body, when left unchecked, creates the perfect breeding ground for the five parasites, or opportunistic invaders, that have the potential to wreak havoc on our health.

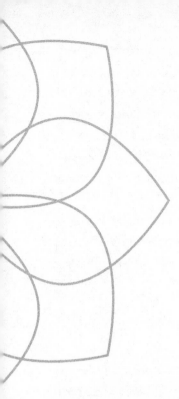

Chapter 3

# The Five Parasites: The Opportunists That Wreak Havoc

The cough that won't go away. The gas, bloating, or constipation that will not resolve, despite changing your diet and cleansing the liver. The psoriasis, rash, or acne that refuses to be subdued no matter what formulas you use or treatments you try. The fatigue, depression, or irritability that endures, even when your family or work circumstances change. Stubborn symptoms like these can be confounding, frustrating, and deeply upsetting, because even when you feel you're taking all the right steps, they can persist—for weeks, months, or even years. Sometimes it can feel like they're taking over your life. Trying to resolve these things can feel like being a participant in a mystery story, finding your way through the dark alone with few clues and a broken flashlight.

I have come to understand that most chronic health issues can be tracked to a group of five parasites that if left unchecked have the potential to wreak havoc. In clinical practice, I find that two out of three patients are troubled by at least one of these invaders, though they often do not know it. Human beings exist in a delicate balance with these tiny but tenacious opportunists; when our resistance to them lessens, they can take advantage and gain the upper hand.

parasites are a potential obstacle for all of us yet are largely over-
, and they do much of their disruptive work invisibly and utterly
pected. While two of the five can sometimes be detected with the
naked eye, the others cannot be seen. And because we don't know to
look for them when we feel unwell, doctors frequently don't test for
all the culprits or consider them in their diagnoses. Which means that
these disturbances go largely undiscovered, becoming the root cause of
chronic disease.

The subject of parasites can make us squirm—who really wants to
talk about worm larvae or amoebic infection? But it is essential to bring
it to light, for it can be life-changing to identify these parasites that are
living within us in an unbalanced relationship.

## Uncovering Parasitic Activity

The word *parasite* is defined as an organism that lives on or in another organism and benefits by deriving nutrients at the host's expense. The term
may conjure a tapeworm or roundworm residing in the gut. Worms are
quite common visitors to our bodies—they don't, as is widely assumed,
bother only our furry four-legged friends—yet they are only one of a
group of organisms that engage in parasitic activity. More widespread
than worms are microscopic parasites like an amoeba such as giardia
found in water. Worms and microscopic parasites are responsible for an
enormous amount of the chronic digestive distress like IBS and colitis
that causes suffering for so many.

The third parasites are the group of fungi that includes candida,
which can cause constipation, foggy thinking, rashes, depression, bloating, and sugar cravings. (Environmental mold can cause the same symptoms as candida, as well as lung and respiratory problems that are very
often misdiagnosed as allergies.) The fourth group are viruses—such as
Epstein-Barr, herpes simplex, and herpes zoster—that, even in the absence of pronounced physical symptoms, can exhaust our whole bodies,
cause nerve pain, and bring our spirit and will down. The fifth group is
bacteria, which at a low, chronic level can create swollen joints and at an
acute level can manifest as strep throat, staph infections, food poisoning,

and urinary tract infections. What these five organisms have in common is that after permeating our body, they survive by living off our energy, using it to flourish and reproduce; in all five groups their mode of existence is *parasitic,* or dependent on a host.

In the early eighties, I worked closely with Dr. Parcells to refine my work in medical radiesthesia and deepen my knowledge of parasites and environmental pollution. Viruses like HIV and Epstein-Barr were very much in the public consciousness, though few people outside of specialty medicine understood them; and the depleting effects of parasites were not on the mainstream radar. Yet these parasites, including bacteria, worms, and microscopic parasites, kept showing up as blocks to the flow of subtle energy and as disturbances throughout their tissues, organs, and systems. Just like the interferences from pollution, these parasites could be detected through the frequency of their energy fields. Subtle instruments could detect their presence as an incoherent pattern of energy sometimes weeks before a follow-up test of a blood, urine, or stool sample indicated that anything was amiss.

Finding a parasite often is the significant key to unraveling the mystery of malaise, persistent fatigue, or a full-blown cascade of symptoms that in many cases had been causing suffering but doggedly eluding explanation. Treating the parasite once it was found could feel nothing short of miraculous for someone who'd been unwell for too long. After slowly and gradually clearing the invaders using natural, noninvasive protocols, patients would often report that they felt like their reserves had been unlocked and their vitality, clarity, and optimism had been given back to them. Meanwhile, the uncomfortable issues that had been plaguing them, whether in their belly, sinuses, blood-sugar balance, or state of mind and mood (or elsewhere entirely, for there are no limitations to the parasites' reach in the body) began finally to improve. This understanding grew to be a pillar of Harmonic Healing; without attending to parasites that have taken control of our inner environment, healing was blocked.

The five parasites have been part of the human story throughout time, and their capacity to make us ill is quite well known. Ingest some water contaminated with giardia, and you will experience violent diarrhea—

known to vacationers as the dreaded "Montezuma's revenge"—as your body attempts to expel the parasite; become infected with the flu virus, and your body will initiate fever and vomiting to try to clear it from the system. Acute incidents like these convince us that when exposures to these parasites occur, we know about it beyond a shadow of a doubt. After the worst has passed, we tend to assume that the infecting agents have died off; our body is once again restored to a state of balance.

But through studying thousands of patients, it is clear that this is not always the case. Even parasites like worms, which we imagine to be unpleasant and obvious, don't always make a dramatic entry or exit; infection by these stealthy invaders can create negligible symptoms, or no symptoms at all. Furthermore, when an acute case of worms, amoebic infection, or any other parasite *does* occur and a treatment appears to heal it, the offending invader is not necessarily banished from the body—it is simply suppressed and reduced in numbers or power. The activity diminishes to a level that we may not necessarily notice, but the parasite and its potential for disruption may still be there.

Time after time I have observed that a crucial factor determines whether a parasite becomes active and disruptive enough to trigger a downward spiral of health or stays dormant and submissive, without causing any trouble to body or mind. That factor is the balance of the body's electromagnetic field and the strength of the vital force.

### The Five Parasites

You don't pick up parasites only when traveling overseas—though that certainly can be the source, as anyone who has been hit by diarrhea in a developing country will agree! And they don't come only from exposure to extremely unhygienic conditions like eating out of dirty kitchens and enjoying street food, surfing after a rainstorm has washed effluvia into the ocean, or tending to homes and landscapes hit by floodwaters. These scenarios will certainly make infection more likely, but the reality is that we're exposed to parasites in mundane ways every day. Eating contaminated foods, walking barefoot in a vegetable patch or park, or sleeping in a bed with a pet that has parasites are the common-or-garden ways that parasites can make contact with our bodies. It never ceases to surprise patients when I ask them if they've been swimming in a lake over the summer or been dining on sushi—both these innocuous activities can expose us to parasites that we never see, smell, taste, or feel.

The parasites are a diverse group; once they infect us, whether through food, water, a bite, sexual contact, or the skin, they can take up residence not only in our intestines, which is where worms, microscopic parasites, and candida tend to first make their mark, but also in the liver, lungs, brain, and other organs, as well as the lymphatic system and blood. The symptoms that the body creates in response to them can vary widely depending on where the parasites are living and causing their damage. Yet even within this wide range of possibilities, there is considerable overlap in the symptoms created by this group. All five types of parasite create inflammation by stimulating ongoing immune system responses—either by registering as an invader in the body or by allowing foreign particles to get through the gut wall—and they typically cause fatigue as the body's energy reserves are used to fuel a nonstop process of resistance. Further clues suggesting the presence of parasites:

- Ongoing digestive distress, including diarrhea, constipation, bloating, gas, and bad breath, as well as syndromes diagnosed as IBS and colitis, that do not clear up through dietary improvements and a restorative liver-cleansing program like the one in this book. Food sensitivities can also be caused by parasites living in the intestines and triggering immune system responses to certain foods, as they colonize and irritate the gut wall and contribute to gut permeability.

- Skin issues like eczema, psoriasis, and rashes, as well as acne (including cystic acne) and skin bumps, which can result when the parasites excrete their waste products into the bloodstream and the body works to eliminate them through its biggest detoxification organ, the skin. Boils and skin infections, meanwhile, indicate the activity of bacteria or a parasite in the lymph system. Rosacea can be caused by bacteria in the blood.
- Brain fog, depression, sleep disturbance, and more complex neurological issues, which can be caused by one or more parasites.
- Weight loss and malnourishment, which can arise when parasites living in the intestines block the proper absorption of food; weight gain and difficulty losing unwanted weight can arise from undiagnosed parasites disrupting normal metabolic and detoxification function, no matter what diet you are on.
- Prediabetic and diabetic activity, which can be the result of parasites infecting areas of the pancreas and surrounding tissues, interfering with glucose and insulin metabolism.

Another thing these five parasites have in common? They operate mainly out of sight. While the fungus candida's overgrowth can be perceived when you know what to look for, and an extreme case of worms may be visible in the stool, by and large we do not perceive the evidence of parasites. Testing will typically help to identify them, but it is important to note that many tests—such as the standard ones for worms and microscopic parasites—fail to find the parasites at low-grade levels of chronic activity. (Worm larvae, for example, are so minuscule that they typically evade detection, making it important to use a treatment that clears the dormant larvae in the mucous lining, as well as the active worms.)

## 1. MICROSCOPIC PARASITES

These are so small they cannot be seen with the naked eye. They include giardia from water contaminated by animal or human feces; flukes, microscopic worms which can come from snails living at the bottom of lakes or brackish waters; *Entamoeba histolytica,* transmitted through contaminated food and water; filaria, transmitted by sand-flea bites; and, very important, the Lyme spirochete, transmitted by a deer tick and, as we currently understand it, also through sexual contact and from mother to child in utero. Note that several of these are considered by modern science to be bacteria; after forty years of measuring the energy of parasites, I have observed these to read energetically as the category I call microscopic parasites and from an energetic standpoint it is important to treat them as such. (See Lyme Syndrome, page 76).

**SOURCES OF EXPOSURE:** Contaminated salad bars, undercooked or raw meat or fish, unhygienic home kitchen and restaurant settings; drinking contaminated water; swimming in ponds, lakes, and rivers; mosquito, flea, and tick bites that release organisms into the bloodstream.

**SYMPTOMS:** Diarrhea, smelly stools, weight loss, joint pain, dark circles under the eyes, adrenal exhaustion, poor and restless sleep, neurological disturbances, nerve pain and itching around the rectum, and the swelling of limbs known as elephantiasis, caused by filarial infection from a sand-flea bite affecting the lymph system. Liver flukes, typically ingested by swallowing lake water, are an often-undiagnosed cause of liver stress and can cause liver cysts. Skin rashes can be caused by these microscopic parasites colonizing the bloodstream and releasing toxins into the lymph system.

## 2. WORMS

Often visible to the naked eye, these include hookworms, tapeworms, threadworms, ropeworms, and roundworms such as *Ascaris lumbricoides,* which move through our organs and tissues and have an affinity for the lungs.

**SOURCES OF EXPOSURE:** Travel; unwashed produce; raw fish and undercooked meat, particularly pork (the worms may or may not be visible and the larvae are hidden); walking barefoot on soil (such as an organic garden in which chemicals have not killed off hookworms) or on grass contaminated with animal feces; close contact with animals that are infected and transmit through licking; cross-contamination between adults and children in preschool environments (in the case of pinworms, a type of threadworm).

**SYMPTOMS:** Worms can take up residence in the intestines, where they can interfere with digestion, create constipation and/or an itchy rectum, and cause poor absorption of nutrients, leading to fatigue, anemia, weight loss, and bad breath. (A clue that a child has worms is a trio of symptoms: scratching their rear end, picking their nose, and grinding their teeth at night, all due to the nocturnal irritation that worms cause, including laying itchy eggs around the rectum.) Pancreatic and gallbladder problems can also arise from worms living near the pancreatic and bile ducts. Depression, poor or restless sleep, or nightmares can also occur due to the nocturnal worm activity. Respiratory troubles in the lungs and sinuses, including asthma, can come from *Ascaris lumbricoides,* aka roundworms, a tissue parasite that can spread to the lungs. Trichinella spiralis is a worm commonly found in pork that can cause digestive distress and sulfurous gas, then migrate to tissues where it can cause cysts. (Trichinosis is the infection caused by this roundworm.)

## 3. FUNGI

This category includes candida, a yeast that grows in moist interiors of the body such as the intestines and vagina, as well as household molds that can proliferate in buildings and on foods that can colonize the lungs and sinus cavities. Molds and yeast can also colonize and affect brain tissue. Mold toxins block the detoxification of heavy metals; when mold is present, the effects of metals in the body are amplified and made worse.

SOURCES OF EXPOSURE: Fungi such as candida exist naturally in the intestines (in small amounts and in balance with other flora in the gut) but can proliferate dramatically after antibiotic use, from elevated exposure to interferences and stress, and when the diet includes significant amounts of sugar and yeast. Household mold can proliferate especially in older homes and humid climates.

SYMPTOMS: Candida and other yeasts reveal themselves through multiple symptoms: bloating and constipation caused by gut dysbiosis, the overgrowth of candida and yeast in the gut; a thick white coating on the tongue; vaginal discharge; dandruff; and rashes (particularly those that itch). Fungus under the toenails is another clear indicator, as are sugar and dairy cravings, depression, brain fog, emotional instability, and wakefulness between 1:00 and 3:00 A.M. Candida releases water as it builds up in the colon and can also cause edema, or generalized swelling, and also contributes to problems losing extra weight.

## 4. VIRUSES

The most commonly detected viruses are Epstein-Barr, herpes simplex and herpes zoster, cytomegalovirus (CMV), and HIV. Some viruses, like the flu virus, can largely clear out of our bodies but can leave toxins that exist for years. Viruses can affect all organs and systems but are especially connected to our nervous system.

**SOURCES OF EXPOSURE:** Viruses can be airborne, transmitted through sexual contact or in utero, and injected into our blood through vaccines such as those for polio, chicken pox, and flu. Viruses remain in our bodies for our lifetime and carry over to future generations.

**SYMPTOMS:** Fatigue; shooting pains; nerve sensations; loss of will, including depression; other neurological symptoms such as ringing in the ears and paralysis; and canker sores, also known as fever blisters or herpes vesicles, in the mouth and other orifices are indicators of viral infection. Acute cases of illness like shingles can occur, or diseases related to a low-functioning immune system, as in mononucleosis and HIV.

Viruses are difficult to overcome; they create a code on the cells that remains with us. We want the virus to become latent or inactive and live in harmony with us.

## 5. BACTERIA

This group includes the most common bacteria that live in our systems, such as streptococci, staphylococci, and the tuberculosis bacteria (that some of us are born with, as the frequency of the bacteria can be passed down through generations and remain in our DNA. Homeopaths know to look for the "tubercular miasm" in these cases, a piece of information that helps to understand the patient's constitution).

**SOURCES OF EXPOSURE:** We may already have these bacteria living quietly in our systems; external sources can include food that has gone bad, contaminated water, or contamination from another person carrying an infection.

**SYMPTOMS:** Inflammation of all sorts; pain and swelling in joints; rashes; boils; rheumatoid arthritis; fever and fatigue; food poisoning; infections, including respiratory and blood infections; bloating; nausea; stomach ulcers; and UTIs and bladder infections are just a few of the symptoms that bacteria can cause.

Not everyone has to attend to parasites through targeted protocols in order to feel well, because restoring vitality and clearing interferences can often be enough to help the body keep them in check. But awareness that they might be a cause of chronic conditions, whether now or in the future, would be an investigation into their symptoms. With the awareness of them, we can bring them out of the shadows and start to ask better questions sooner rather than later, and connect the dots when we are not feeling well. If required, we can take positive steps to reduce their hold on us and avoid unnecessary suffering since symptoms from one parasite can be similar to those induced by another, identifying the root cause is not always a one-step process and can require dedication and time.

## Interferences and Opportunists: A Lasting Relationship

We cannot live sequestered from parasites or isolate ourselves from their reach. Worms, microscopic parasites, fungi, bacteria, and viruses are around us at all times, and to varying degrees and they are always *within* us as well. They are part of our ecosystem.

These parasites can be so extensive that I screen my patients regularly. What I am looking for is not black or white—the absolute presence or nonpresence of a parasite. Health works more subtly than that. Our well-being is not predicated on whether a parasite exists within us or not but rather on whether the conditions in our body are such that we are allowing them to *take over*. Dealing with parasites involves a shift in thinking from what we've been taught to believe: Our challenge is not necessarily to banish them but to exist in harmony with them so they do not interfere with our vital force, disrupting our balance of health.

Over my years of treating people with extremely diverse lifestyles, from globe-trotters who visit the corners of the world to stay-at-home parents intimate with preschool germs, I have observed a striking commonality: When our body's electromagnetic field is balanced, the incidence of parasites gaining the upper hand and negatively impacting our health is dramatically reduced. In the opposite scenario, when the energy field has become weakened, imbalanced, and blocked, the opposite result occurs; parasitic infection is more common and its enduring and chronic power is heightened.

This is because there is an affinity between parasitic activity and energetic incoherence—an interdependent relationship of sorts. Parasites are drawn to the strong fields of heavy metals and chemicals, like birds to bread crumbs, because an accumulation of pollution and stress changes the environment of the body at the cellular level and makes it a more welcoming and supportive place for them to live. The parasites resonate with the frequencies of heavy metals and chemicals; low frequency is the frequency of disease activity, and when the metals accumulate, the natural immunity is challenged and parasites can proliferate. Simultaneously, the aggravating fields of radiation suppress the immune and nervous systems, further creating an environment that parasites like. Instead of being a well-protected kingdom, therefore, the body becomes a welcoming host. It transmits the message "The gates are open, defenses are down, come on in and make yourself at home!"

From my observation, heavy metals, chemicals, radiation, stress, and shock are the predictable precursors to the welcoming of parasites: When a parasite like a worm or candida has taken hold in the system and we peel back the layers of the onion, we discover that metals, chemicals, and radiation are proliferating underneath, making the symptoms the parasite creates persistent and hard to resolve. Though our healing mechanisms normally strive to repel invaders and protect us from their effects, when the pollution persists, its stronger field wins. The metals and chemicals resonate with parasites, creating an attraction that invites the invaders in the body and makes them much more challenging to neutralize.

From this place, a vicious cycle can begin: As the parasites gain ground in a weakened body, sustaining themselves and reproducing off our resources, they create chronic inflammation. This mobilizes the body's defenses; it digs into its healing reserves to maintain balance. If the reserves are already depleted from a weakened field, the efforts to resist the parasites take a toll on the body, stealing energy that is required for daily needs. For already exhausted adrenal glands, using up the reserves in this way can be the straw that breaks the camel's back. It contributes to a cascade of chronic symptoms that can get worse in times of stress and weaken the healing potential further still. Making things trickier is the fact that when left unacknowledged and untreated, the parasites can begin to exist in combination, with one creating a hospitable environment for the others. Worms, microscopic parasites, and candida excrete waste material that in turn creates bacteria. A bacteria depleting the reserves can make it possible for latent virus to become active and turn into an acute infection. When one parasite flares up, we might look for another behind the scenes.

Once the initial parasite has been neutralized, balanced etheric energy and a strong vital force will very often keep the parasites in check.

But we never fully banish or destroy the parasites. These opportunists tend to remain in the body at a vibrational level: After treating candida overgrowth, there will likely still be fungus in the system; after clearing worms and microscopic parasites, larvae may remain and hatch at a later date; and in the case of viruses, they never leave us entirely and at best remain dormant in our system.

What we want is for parasites to stay dormant and unable to tip the balance of energy in their favor, so that we can enjoy health. This occurs as long as the vital force is nourished and the etheric energy is flowing because health is a balance of body, mind, emotions, and spirit.

In allopathic medicines disease is understood to originate from the pathogen. In subtle medicine, we look at the environment that the parasite inhabits as the causative factor and understand that if it is corrected, the disease activity can resolve and the body can rebalance. From this perspective, the parasites actually become a gauge of our current state of health; they are like our watchdogs. When one or more of them flares up from a dormant phase and becomes active, it can be a clue that the conditions within have become out of balance; it is time to put a little more effort into eating good foods, clearing toxins, reducing stress, resting more, supporting our vital force, and, if needed, doing a program of treatment to put them back in their place. It can also offer another type of clue, alerting us that we have fallen out of balance mentally and emotionally and are vulnerable in an area of our psyche.

If we look more deeply at the purpose of these parasites, we realize that they are only here to bring us awareness—of our individual nature, of our strengths and weaknesses, and of our current state of health. Though they test us with adversity, they invite us to make shifts in how we live and wake us up to live in accordance with our true nature. The parasites, as challenging as they can be, play an unseen role of keeping us connected to what is happening within. When they are viewed this way, a space of relief, and healing, can open. Many of my Lyme patients have learned that they can manage the extent to which spirochetes can take over their body—and even get the spirochetes to become dormant and inactive—through healthy practices. As the patient's commitment to self-care increases with the acknowledgment that the optimum level of health is one of balance, it can be incredible how in a short time much of the pain associated with the Lyme syndrome can melt away.

## THE SYNERGY OF INTERFERENCES AND OPPORTUNISTS

The relationship between environmental interferences and opportunists can play out in many ways. When we travel, the elevated presence of heavy metals in the air and in food, makes us especially susceptible to picking up parasites from the food or water. The stomach acid can get suppressed by metals and falls too low to be the reliable "first line of defense" against food-borne parasites that it is meant to be. I recommend to take baths before trips and give a homeopathic remedy to counter-act metals inhaled and ingested while traveling; those who follow these steps experience far fewer incidences of parasites. It's not just travelers to other third world countries who take extra protective steps to maintain their health; many people "pick something up" after any air travel, and this is partly because of the heightened exposure to radiation in flight, as well as the general stress of travel, disturbs the balance of the electromagnetic field, making us more vulnerable to parasites like bacteria and viruses. Taking a detoxifying bath soon after a flight is one way to support our body's resilience in these moments.

For those who already know they have parasites entrenched in their system but have yet to find treatments that make them better, the answer almost always comes down to unresolved interferences and shock. When treating patients infected with the spirochete that causes the Lyme syndrome, elevated levels of heavy metals like mercury, aluminum, and lead are always found. Neutralizing the effects of the metals is as vital as attending to the parasite; only when the field has been brought into balance can the body begin the process of letting go of the spirochete.

The same dynamic can occur around unresolved shock. A parasite that has gone dormant and ceased to cause problems can be reactivated in a period of high stress or shock, as well as after a traumatic event. One patient had resolved her persistent parasite problems after setting healthy boundaries on a troubling family relationship; several years later, when she finally visited the family member in question, she experienced an immediate return of symptoms. (This woman was so familiar with doing her parasite-clearing programs that she restored order quite quickly, then reexamined the boundaries she had set in the relationship.) We cannot expect to heal our bodies from parasites without addressing the interferences and shock; the interferences and opportunists that exist hand in hand, and the environment we live in.

## Harmonic Healing and Parasites: A Multidimensional Look

Nothing in health is ever purely physical. The presence and activity of parasites in our bodies can be better understood when we see them in a holistic way and as connected to our individual natures. The same parasite does not express in the same way in every person; we all have our own tendencies toward hosting certain ones over others. One person tends to get food poisoning more often; another struggles with persistent candida; yet another with asthmatic episodes originating in roundworm infection. Over time we can get to know our individual tendencies and notice early on when parasites may flare up.

The prism through which I understand this individual interaction with the five parasites is the five elements, the foundational components of nature that combine to form the matter of our bodies, our personality or individual nature, and the ways we think and what we feel. Water governs the realm of emotions; fire governs the processes of transformation, metabolism, and defense. Through decades of clinical work, study, and research, I have come to see each parasite as connected to one of the elements—earth, water, fire, air, ether—and this connection can be observed not only in the physical part of the body that the parasite disturbs but also in the types of disturbances to the mental and emotional fields it provokes.

In yoga and Ayurveda, the number five is the organizing factor of life. From the genesis of the five elements, we have five senses, five fingers, and five predominant tastes. In life and in health, we endeavor to maintain a dance of balance among the five, which are constantly in relationship with one another—for example, by being aware of all five senses as we move through the day and preparing meals that, over the course of a day, stimulate all five tastes. When one of the five becomes overly stimulated or aggravated, or overly weakened, we gently address this through food, through breathing exercises, or through natural remedies, in order to maintain balanced relationship. Addressing imbalances of the elements in order to resolve symptoms and restore health is the heart of many traditional medicines.

When it comes to the parasites, the model of fives has shaped the types of treatments I use. I have found that each parasite is particularly attracted to a weakness in at least one element within us. The weakness could simply be part of our unique design—we all have areas of strength and weakness in our body and psyche—or it could result from lifestyle or stress pushing us out of balance. When there is a weakness in that element, we tend to experience shifts in the ways we feel, function, look, or think.

The model of fives has helped to give a more nuanced picture of *why* we have tendencies toward certain parasites; it has to do with an imbalance in that element within ourselves, which plays out in the five *passions*. The five passions are power, desire, love, wisdom, and will. They are intimately involved with the five parasites, giving us another way into understanding why we may be infected by them. When an element is out of balance, the related *passion* gets out of balance also—it can be either overexpressed or underexpressed. Our behavior shifts to an extreme; we might become more dominating and harsh, or airy and ungrounded, or disconnected from our will. This could be described as the psychospiritual aspect of the five parasites.

This resonance helps us to understand why certain emotions or states of feeling correspond with infection by the culprits; and why harboring a particular emotional state—consciously or not—can make infection with its related parasite more likely or more entrenched. A person who is locked in a personal battle around power might be more susceptible to worms; another person who experiences disappointment, longing, and grief may find themselves working for some time to release stubborn candida. Furthermore, once we are infected, that parasite can amplify the frequency of that emotional state, intensifying our experience of it. Our minds might believe that it is the world out there creating our experience—or something or someone else's fault—when it is the presence of a parasite that is directing how we see and experience our life.

When we become aware of this dynamic, our state of mind, mood, and behavior can sometimes offer a finer-level clue to the unseen stirring of parasitic activity. This can help us to take action early to address the parasite and return to balance. The relationship can be particularly apparent in children, who often display pronounced behavioral shifts—because they don't try to edit or conceal what they are feeling. Mothers who I have worked with have learned that this can be most apparent when their children have a case of worms and volatile power struggles occur along with the itching symptoms described above.

This model also helps us to heal our whole selves. When a parasite is persisting or continuing to occur even after treatments are completed, we can look at whether our outlook and state of mind are contributing to the frequent reoccurrence of the parasite. We can ask not only what treatment we need to do through remedies and diet but also what we may need to change about how we are relating to the world mentally, emotionally, and spiritually. This approach can help us start to find some peace on our healing journey. We may even find that experiencing a parasite has been necessary to help us become aware of patterns in our mental and emotional states that don't serve us, or see our shadow sides and areas of weaknesses and learn how to work with them. Homeopathy, with its ability to attend to our subtle nature, is particularly effective in helping to move through such holistic healing experiences.

Take a look at the parasites through this model, and you may find new clues coming from your watchdog that you are becoming more predisposed to symptoms and conditions that, if left unresolved, could develop into disease.

Claude came to me suffering from a skin rash that had erupted all over his body with no obvious cause. It did not seem to come from food allergies, nor was it related to stress. His doctors were perplexed but prescribed cortisone, an anti-inflammatory steroid, to take down the rash and give him some comfort. Claude did not want to go that route; he knew that cortisone could exhaust the adrenals and that suppressing symptoms in the skin in this way could even cause lung congestion, due to the interrelated nature of the skin and the lungs.

Upon analysis of Claude's blood, I found a resonance of hematobium; after a few questions, we deduced this had occurred during his summer swims in a local lake, during which he had inadvertently swallowed lake water. I told him that the skin rash was the natural response of the body to this invading presence; it was trying to clear it through the skin. In some cases we might experience the body effectively succeeding and the rash subsiding, but Claude needed help to clear it out of the system. He followed the Harmonic Healing program with the addition of the eight-day milk cleanse to clear the microscopic parasite; and by addressing the cause and not just the symptoms, he was able to clear the rash and return to feeling well again.

## FIVE PARASITES, FIVE ELEMENTS, FIVE PASSIONS: AN ALTERNATIVE MODEL OF TREATMENT

**WORMS are connected to the EARTH element,** which governs our self-empowerment and the way we stand our ground. Earth expresses in the center of our body, our digestive and detoxification system. Worms burrow in the soil—which is the medium through which we often get exposed to them—and in similar fashion, they burrow into our body's center.

**PASSION:** Power.

*Imbalance:* Becoming harsh and controlling, ungrounded, undermined, disempowered, or low in self-esteem and energy.

*Treatment:* Herbs from the earth like wormwood, clove, and black walnut. It is important to follow a protocol that clears the unhatched larvae that have been laid in the mucous lining of the intestines by using digestive enzymes. Mucus can build up from undigested protein, which is why tending to the earth element of the body with bowel and liver cleanses, along with food imbued with etheric energy, helps to release worms and mucus.

........................

**MICROSCOPIC PARASITES are connected to the AIR element.** They are imperceptible to the eye, like air; amoebas affect the digestive power and spirochetes can affect our nervous system while releasing bacteria into the blood and the joints—the area where air accumulates in the body.

**PASSION:** Wisdom.

*Imbalance:* Feeling lost, cut off from self-knowledge.

*Treatment:* They function in an anaerobic environment; thus we use oxygenating treatments, such as oxygenating herbs like cayenne.

**FUNGI are connected to the WATER element,** which governs emotions and desires. In the body, it is our fluids that hold our emotions. Fungi thrive in damp and swampy environments.

**PASSION:** Desire.

*Imbalance:* Longing, deprivation, self-pity. Dampness and stagnation in the body can be mirrored by emotions stuck in states of longing for sweetness and love, which can feed a tendency to indulge in sweet foods and drinks. This can make candida especially hard to move out of the body.

*Treatment:* Clearing heavy metals and chemicals, strict liver-cleansing, no-sugar/low-carbohydrate diet, herbal antifungals, and patience.

........................

**BACTERIA are connected to the FIRE element.** They initiate processes of inflammation in the body, including fever and pain. (The heat of rheumatoid arthritis, which is often bacterial in cause, can feel as if the body has a deep inner fever.)

**PASSION:** Love.

*Imbalance:* Feeling angry, irritable, fearful, and "lack of love."

*Treatment:* Homeopathic remedies such as belladonna, *Nat. mur.,* sulfur, and mercurius; a clean, nourishing diet; and blood-cleansing and immune-supportive herbs like echinacea and red clover.

**VIRUSES are connected to the ETHER element.** Like ether, they are so subtle that they often elude detection, which is why viruses are often misdiagnosed or unaddressed. They are also omnipresent like ether; a virus can imprint a viral code on our cells that passes on to future generations.

**PASSION:** Will. Ether is the space and the energy of everything; thus the virus particularly interferes with our will to be.

*Imbalance:* Loss of will, depression, hopelessness.

*Treatment:* Dedicated immune-system and vitality support with food and herbs, good lifestyle practices such as meditation, finding peace in nature, drinking good water, and getting restful sleep; building the will for life through homeopathic treatment, time in nature, and connecting with one's higher nature—which is connected to the ether.

## 5 PARASITES, 5 ELEMENTS, 5 PASSIONS

| Worms | Fungus | Bacteria | Microscopic Parasites | Virus |
|-------|--------|----------|-----------------------|-------|
| Earth | Water | Fire | Air | Ether |
| Power | Desire | Love | Wisdom | Will |

David, an entrepreneur and rare-wine dealer, had been struggling with Lyme syndrome for more than ten years when we first met. Antibiotics had initially helped suppress the symptoms, but in a period of heightened stress, the syndrome came roaring back, rendering him very depleted energetically, exhausted physically, and struggling to get through each day. His mind felt fogged and his energy and zest for life gone. To battle the increasing severity of symptoms, David was given ever-stronger rounds of antibiotics. When these drugs did not work, he began to be very fearful. When I checked his physical-etheric energy, I found significant interference from high levels of mercury; he told me he'd eaten sushi daily, especially tuna. He was also overtaken by candida as a result of his intensive antibiotic treatments, and this was causing brain fog and pain all over his body.

David began the milk cleanse, replete with antiparasitic herbs, to address the spirochete levels, and halfway through the program, he began feeling 75 percent better. Over time he was able to control the spirochetes and get to a place where normal testing was not detecting them at all. I explained to him that even though the tests were negative, the vibration of spirochetes was in his body and suggested that we monitor this occasionally until his vital force came back stronger.

For David, clearing the candida was the hardest part of the healing process; he had to strictly follow a candida diet and completely reevaluate his relationship to indulgences— the wines that were his lifeblood and the high-end dining out that accompanied his business had to be tempered and brought under more control. David gained the awareness that it was the candida that made him feel so poorly and not the Lyme spirochete—even a few sips of wine could bring on a foggy-headed episode. Determined to feel better, David stuck with his diet, and as the candida cleared, his health and his personal mission in life came back into focus.

Today David is proud that the conventional Lyme test through his doctor shows him to be clear of the spirochete, and he is involved with educating others about the lymes syndrome through sharing his personal journey to health. And now he can enjoy his fine wine without overindulging and negative effects.

## Neutralizing Parasites

Making our home inhospitable to parasites by changing the environment through detoxification support and the Liver-Cleansing Program can very often be enough to start to clear up parasitic activity—even if we're not aware that one or more of the five have been bothering us. After improving the environment at the cellular-energy level and restoring our vital force, worms, microscopic parasites, fungus, bacteria, and viruses can begin to resolve. The lessened pollution levels from environmental interference allow the lymph to flow and the immune system to do its work. (If candida has been detected at the outset, and the candida version of the program is followed, significant headway can be made on reducing this parasite as well.) And when we take time to breathe and move oxygen through our bodies, we not only reduce stress but also make the environment less welcoming to the parasites that like anaerobic environments. It is quite common for uncomfortable and persistent problems like bloating, constipation, and skin issues to begin to clear after the six-week program, with continued improvements as the longer-term lifestyle is followed.

In Harmonic Healing, herbal and homeopathic medicine is used to treat the five parasites. This is in contrast to the use of drug regimens to either treat the symptoms or try to destroy the parasite itself; these can be toxic and difficult to use for a long enough time to stop the parasitic activity. Symptoms may resolve temporarily, but then a few months later, they reappear. It is also preferable to clear the candida via natural means, through dietary protocols with herbal antifungals for support. These are effective *if* you stay on them for long enough—often it can take many months to neutralize the candida. Clearing parasites is best done alongside a protocol to clear the heavy metals, chemicals, and radiation. Although all parasites present their own conundrum, natural methods have proven successful to clear them and then help to rebuild the body and create balance—and allow us to see if there is another layer to clear next, such as bacteria or fungus present that may appear after clearing worms.

For nearly four decades, I have used a proprietary protocol for clearing worms and microscopic parasites. In the Light Harmonics 8-day milk cleanse, either goat or cow milk is the medium for carrying into the body herbs that target the parasite. As the milk gently yet persistently draws the worms and microscopic parasites out of their hiding places, a special mix of antiparasitic herbs clears the worms or microscopic parasites so that the body can be free of their influence and begin to rebuild vitality and reserves. The milk cleanse is followed by digestive enzymes such as pepsin, to clear the mucus and larvae that the worms have left behind. This eight-day milk protocol, if followed properly, reliably clears the parasitic activity, including the spirochetes that cause the Lyme syndrome. We then turn to lifting away the next layer of parasitic activity, which is typically candida that may have existed in the intestines for years. The reason that this method is effective is that parasites love milk; it acts as a bait to lure the parasites into the digestive tract, where the antiparasitic herbs can do their work.

As a side note, this affinity with milk is very often the cause of the digestive disturbance many people experience after consuming dairy products—the milk is activating or energizing and feeding parasites in the system. When the parasites are brought under control, the dairy issues can often resolve.

Healing is a process, and in many cases stubborn parasitic conditions have taken years to layer themselves into the body. Relieving the body of their influence and restoring the balance of health will take some time, but if we approach this calmly, patiently, and diligently, we can make it back to our original state, enjoying radiant health and clarity with peace in the mind and body.

Living in harmony means living with a heightened awareness of ourselves; getting to know what our body feels like when it is well and unwell; becoming familiar with our unique tendencies to certain parasites and cultivating an understanding of how they reactivate during periods of heightened stress or vulnerability. There is great power in this awareness; we can take care of ourselves continuously, avoiding falling into states of exhaustion or overwhelm, because that is when symptoms can come racing back. When we live in this awareness, we do not overly fret about parasites, but we simply keep in consideration that if we've treated a parasite once, it's likely that we might have to do so again—and should we start to feel unwell, we know where to look and connect the dots sooner rather than later.

Many patients get in the habit of not only doing Liver-Cleansing Programs on an annual basis but also incorporating parasite cleanses once or twice a year, especially if their lifestyle includes travel overseas, living or working with pets or animals, or eating sushi, pork, or raw vegetables straight out of the garden or from a salad bar. Today there are many formulas available for parasite cleansing that can be used successfully. After all, we deworm our pets regularly, so why not bring that awareness of clearing parasites to ourselves as well? We know that there will always be parasites in our environment, there will frequently be parasites in our body, and we can't always control when our body begins to become imbalanced. What we can take control of is how our body is interacting with these parasites. Even if you have lived with parasites sapping your energy and vitality for some time, everything can begin to change when you start to know, from the core of your being, that your body is your domain, not theirs. From that place of awareness, you begin to become master of yourself.

## Lyme Syndrome: Treating the Spirochete

The Lyme epidemic of the last three decades is one of the most notorious examples of parasitic activity affecting our health, and the epidemic continues to grow. New Lyme sufferers are often seen at our office and are given the milk protocol that they've heard about with good results. And many long-term patients find that at some point they are exposed to and infected by spirochetes. I have also been infected twice by spirochetes and know firsthand the devastating feeling that accompanies the exposure.

The spirochete is still something of a mystery in medical science, and it evades a definitive understanding. It is quite widely described as a bacterium because the antibodies to bacteria are clearly shown in the blood. The patient is therefore typically treated with strong antibiotics in the attempt to stop the Lyme syndrome. For many people this strategy only temporarily subdues symptoms, and resurgences of the syndrome continue; they become confused, demoralized, and weakened by this intense assault on their system. I have come to know the spirochete in a different way. The energy field of the spirochete reads as a *microscopic parasite* and therefore I treat it as such, using oxygenating herbs with the milk cleanse. The bacteria that are present in the blood are the *waste products* of this microscopic parasite, and what I have learned is that we cannot clear the bacteria and coinfections until the spirochete itself is dealt with—in my approach through the milk-cleanse protocol, along with detoxifying baths to neutralize heavy metals, radiation, and chemicals. As the spirochetes begin to diminish, so do the bacterial waste and the resulting inflammation it causes.

The treatment does not usually stop there. While dealing with spirochetes is relatively straightforward for many patients, many of them then undertake the longer and more challenging phase of treatment, which involves clearing candida that has usually taken over the intestines after months, or even years, of powerful antibiotic treatment that has significantly altered the gut flora. With patience, results come. By clearing the spirochetes and candida, and following a lifestyle of gentle detoxification and good nourishment through well-chosen food, many Lyme patients report good results in clearing this syndrome.

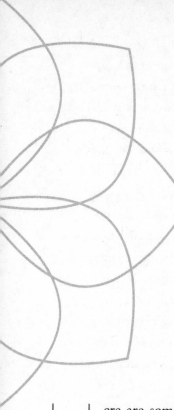

Chapter 4

# Digest Your Food, Digest Your Life: Restoring the Power of the Liver

H ere are some of the things that our liver, our most important organ of digestion and detoxification, deals with daily. The complex combinations of foods in our daily meals, including the unnatural fats they contain—or the natural fats eaten in unnatural amounts. The stimulants we might sip to wake up and the pills we might take to relax. And more: The problems we mull over, trying to solve, and the emotions that churn through us, simply as part of being human, are also processed by the liver. Our liver is the *mediator* that exists between us and the world; everything that comes into us must go through it in some way in order to be transformed—then either absorbed and used or neutralized and released. The responsibilities of the liver are significant and broad.

Yet we rarely consider the state of our liver or link it to how we feel— beyond, perhaps, noting that it took a hit the morning after a big night out. Even though the liver is always giving us clues to its condition, we don't always connect the dots. When we feel energized upon waking and enjoy glowing skin, bright eyes, and a clear mind, we might not realize that our liver is probably quite happy and getting much of what it needs to do its work. Should we feel sluggish and slowed down, bloated, puffy, or constipated, however, or should we notice problem skin in the mirror or suffer frequent headaches and nausea or bad PMS or hot flashes, or if we feel stuck in low spirits or are quick to explode with anger . . . we'd be wise to understand that the signs are telling us that our liver is congested and our lymphatics—the drainage system that works in tandem with the liver to keep us cleansed—are getting overburdened and need some TLC.

In other times and cultures, checking the functioning of the liver was seen as pivotal in order to know how the body was detoxifying. Similarly the lymph system, which is known as the system of longevity in Ayurveda, was also observed, to see if the lymph was stagnant as a result of poor liver function. (Because stagnation in the lymph system is so common, many of the poses and practices in yoga address it.) The liver has long been seen as the linchpin around which energy, vitality, metabolic balance, hormone balance, reproductive health, and a radiant appearance revolve. It also has a powerful impact on mental clarity and emotional stability and, taking the ripple effect to subtler levels still, our sense of purpose in life.

The typical liver today is weak, congested, and overworked. A liver in this state cannot efficiently metabolize or absorb food because toxins are accumulating in the blood and tissues, causing congestion in the lymph system. This congestion is the result of living in a sea of interferences from environmental pollution, eating poor-quality foods, and mediating the overwhelming stream of information and stimulation that comes before our eyes—much of it, unfortunately, hard to bear and challenging to digest, with bad news circulated more widely than good. And all this performed *without* the protective natural ingredients from Mother Earth and the traditional rhythmic routines of eating, sleeping, and unwinding that would support the liver while it clocks its relentless overtime. In just the same way that *we* get exhausted with too much on our plate and not enough help to get it done, so does our liver.

When we are having indigestion or are fatigued or even irritated, we might first look to the liver. We can learn to catch the signs early by becoming more conscious of the liver's many roles and its fairly simple needs, and then we can learn to attend to it with straightforward measures. Awareness of the liver is the third pillar of restoring our vitality and unlocking our innate healing potential, alongside neutralizing environmental interferences and parasites. As the area in the body where the element of fire resides, it holds our *activating* power, and because it helps to digest food for vitality and for repair, cleanses the blood of impurities and poisons, balances the hormones, and helps to resist and clear parasites, and because it is also our connection point to the subtlest yet most powerful aspect of our innate healing potential—our mental will—I see the liver as our body's most important source due to its innate healing force.

Consider that the word *live* is embedded in this organ's very name. The liver has an unusual capacity for self-repair and regeneration—its ability to regrow is quite legendary, which is why there is a high rate of success in liver transplant operations. The liver asks only that we practice giving it some love and support—when we do this through periodic cleansing and a conscious lifestyle, our liver will love us back.

## Say Hello to Your Liver

Place one hand on your body under your right rib cage and notice a sensation of warmth under your hand. Tucked below the diaphragm and across from the stomach, and weighing about three pounds or more, the large, triangular liver is one of five vital organs that are essential for existence (the other four being the heart, brain, kidneys, and lungs). All your blood passes through it via two different entry points—one coming from the circulatory system and one from the intestinal tract—filled with dissolved nutrients ready for final processing and waste and toxins for detoxifying. At any given time, the liver holds the greatest volume of blood of any organ.

No organ acts alone; the liver occupies the center of the body with the other organs of digestion—the stomach, its small but very important sibling organ the gallbladder, which sits just behind it, and the pancreas,* a gland with which it works in order to oversee the storage and use of blood sugar. Together these digestive organs, which work to extract the heat of energy from food, compose our digestive force. Digestion is the process of turning food into its component chemicals so that the body can use them for fuel, building, and repair. From a multidimensional perspective on health, the act of *digestion* involves more than "breaking down" food; it includes the processing of thoughts and emotions as well. So we take care of this transforming force within us, safeguarding it and giving it what it needs to work its best, knowing it holds the power not only to *digest our food but also to digest our life.* Let me explain.

In subtle medicine we see the digestive force as the power that resides in the body's central wheel of energy, called the *solar* plexus chakra. It is no coincidence that "solar" is the descriptive word here. The sun gives our earth the heat without which life could not exist, and it also gives us the light to see. The solar plexus chakra is similar for us; it is *our seat of vitality,* which is ablaze with the element of fire. It is also our center of purification, cleansing the blood not only so that physical toxins do not accumulate and cause us harm but also so that the life-giving fluid can resonate with etheric energy that vitalizes our body and connects our physical and subtle fields.

Over decades of clinical practice, I have observed that the causes of disharmony and disease can lie in the physical body, the etheric body, the emotional body, or the mental body. It can also lie in the disconnect from the spiritual fields of our higher nature. This means we look at organ function through a multidimensional lens. Understanding the balance of health is like looking at a cobweb of possible connections between the physical and the subtle fields. Is the physical body influencing the subtle fields, or is an emotional or mental block influencing the physical organs through the etheric field? For a practitioner who is trained in subtle medicine, when we look at the liver through the viewpoint of the solar plexus chakra, it can feel as if several lenses are stacked on top of it, each one refracting light onto the next. A chakra is a bridge for energy to move between the physical and the subtle; in the solar plexus chakra, the actions of *digesting, heating, illuminating, and clarifying* are not just physical acts; they are subtle ones too. How well or poorly the organs do their jobs affects the way you function, think, and feel, even your sense of who you are and why you are here. To make this more simple, we can look at the liver through three lenses of the physiological, the subtle, and the supersubtle or esoteric functioning of the liver and see it as the Factory, the Fire, and the Filter.

Betsy, a yoga teacher in New York, was a mother of three who felt she was doing everything she could to be healthy. Yet she suffered from chronic migraines that occurred every three to four weeks, often causing her to lose days of her life as she lay miserably in a darkened room. The rest of the month she suffered from low energy on a daily basis and sometimes dragged herself to work, smiling on the surface but silently berating herself for being so weak. Her doctors couldn't offer resolution to her struggles.

Her evaluation revealed that her liver was sluggish and weak and that, despite her thoughtful vegetarian diet, she was not absorbing adequate nutrition and energy. There was incoherence in her subtle fields; as a mother to teenagers who didn't acknowledge how hard she worked to care for them, Betsy had some anger and resentment yet hadn't allowed herself to feel these "bad" feelings, and consequently her emotional body revealed many unprocessed emotions.

I explained that the stagnation in her liver was contributing to a buildup of pressure and heat in the body; furthermore, her tired liver was not efficiently breaking down used-up hormones and her hormone balance was impaired. Unbeknownst to her, these were the root causes of her headaches. Relieved, Betsy followed the Liver-Cleansing Program, and also embraced homeopathic remedies to help dissolve the unprocessed anger and resentment in her mental field.

As Betsy's liver got a chance to rest and restore, and her body began better absorbing the energy from good food, her liver became more efficient at detoxifying and regulating hormones. After her first three weeks on the Liver-Cleansing Diet, she noticed her headaches had disappeared almost completely; she stayed on her liver-cleansing program, eager to peel away the layers of stress and interference, with the help of homeopathic and Bach Flower remedies, and therapeutic baths. Over time, Betsy was able to make her way to a place she had previously thought unreachable—a world without migraines.

## The Physiology of the Liver: The "Factory"

The textbook understanding of the liver is as the largest chemical factory in the body, responsible for creating the numerous natural chemicals and initiating the processes the body needs to stay nourished, cleansed, and balanced. The liver is an organ with specific vital functions and also secretes chemicals used by other parts of the body. Even though food particles don't pass through the liver like they do through the stomach and the small intestine, it plays a key role in ensuring that the food we ingest can be assimilated. It emulsifies fats in the small intestine into small droplets through the production of bile, a thick, yellow-green digestive juice that gets stored in the gallbladder until needed, then squirted through ducts to the intestine when fatty foods are present. The emulsified drops of fat can then be turned by pancreatic enzymes into fatty acids, which are used as slow-burning fuel, for making hormones (the fatty acid cholesterol is a precursor of hormones, making it essential to physical functioning), and supporting brain and nerve function. With the help of the pancreas, the liver also turns quick-burning glucose dissolved in the blood from carbohydrates into its storable form, glycogen, and then holds on to it until our cells need to burn it for fuel. Meanwhile, if we ingest fructose (the form of sugar naturally found in fruit, in half of sucrose, or table sugar, molecules, and in artificial, corn-derived fructose syrups), the liver will metabolize this also, because cells in the body actually do not use fructose. The liver also breaks down the ethanol in the alcohol we drink.

And after the pancreatic juices turn partly digested proteins in the small intestine into amino acids that dissolve into the bloodstream, the liver finishes the job of protein metabolism too, so that these vital building blocks can be used to repair our tissues and muscles. In addition, the liver stores vitamins A, D, E, K, and $B_{12}$, as well as iron and copper, in a repository of precious reserves that the body needs for many tasks. And all this while creating enzymes that control functions all over the body, including maintaining our body temperature in partnership with the thyroid.

At night when we sleep, the liver performs another set of critical functions. It takes unwanted chemicals out of circulation. This includes hormones that the body has produced and now needs to expel, such as used-up estrogen, along with thyroid and stress hormones and bilirubin from worn-out red blood cells, which helps the cells to transport oxygen. We don't want these things to accumulate; hormones need to exist at proper homeostatic levels in order for us to stay well (estrogen, if it accumulates, can disrupt the thyroid and the gallbladder and contribute to toxicity). When we talk about "balanced hormones," even if what we're looking at is reproductive health or thyroid health, we need to always include the liver in the conversation.

In addition to the internally produced waste matter, *externally* derived chemicals and heavy metals from the environment and our foods, personal-care and cleaning products, indoor atmosphere, and pharmaceutical drugs are also processed by the liver so that they don't become toxic free radicals in the body. If not cleared, these highly reactive molecules can damage cells, suppress the immune system, and make us look and feel older than we are. To avoid this, the liver converts them from fat-soluble forms into water-soluble forms that can be eliminated through the urine or passed back into the intestines and excreted in the stool. If this process of detoxification didn't occur, the accumulating toxins could get easily stored in our fat cells, in our brain, and our nerve sheaths and eventually cause weight gain and dysfunction, or could continue to circulate in the bloodstream and make us feel tired, old, sick, and in pain.

And there is more. Immune cells in the liver's sinusoid tissues help to remove bacteria and viruses that might have made it through the intestinal wall into the bloodstream and prevent them from entering the circulatory system at large, where they could cause real trouble. Meanwhile, the bile that squirts into the intestines to emulsify fat also fulfills a detergent-like function; it sweeps unwanted substances like parasites, along with the detoxified chemicals, used-up bilirubin and hormones, and metals like mercury, aluminum, and lead, out of the body by binding them into the stool. Never underestimate the power of bile! For bile *also* keeps levels of bacteria in the intestinal tract low, helping to prevent inflammation of the intestinal wall that could degrade it and allow pathogens and undigested food particles to cross through it and stimulate a hyperimmune response.

You can probably appreciate by now how a healthy liver, full of energy to digest and detoxify and producing bile in proper amounts, is an important ally not only in allowing us to digest food—the source of subtle energy that nourishes us—but also in resisting and overcoming the five parasites, and unwanted autoimmune responses.

To complete this inventory of impressive feats, the liver also helps to create a very significant amount of lymph, a fluid that plays a critical yet often-overlooked role in nourishment, cleansing, and immunity—so much so that it deserves the same dedicated care we bring to our liver.

## The Liver in Subtle Anatomy: The "Fire"

To appreciate how the condition of the liver affects us in the subtle fields of thought and emotion, it helps to become more familiar with its fire. When I feel a patient's Ayurvedic pulse to assess the balance of the elements of air, fire, and water in their body, if the liver has gotten overburdened, the *pitta* or fire-dominant pulse builds up in intensity and practically jumps out of the skin, indicating that some investigation into the patient's subtle energy, as well as diet, lifestyle, and stress levels, is needed for rebalance. The reverse can also occur: After prolonged toxicity in the liver, the *pitta* pulse can be diminished to the point it can barely be read, indicating a lack of fire.

The element of fire exists to be an activating force. Known in

Ayurveda as *agni,* it is the sacred fire of transformation that resides in the liver. Since the strength or weakness of this fire controls how efficiently we burn and store our fuel, we consider it to be the fire of our digestion. When it comes to weight loss and blood-sugar balance, the liver is where we put our attention first—it can "fire up" the digestive force.

Yet "fire" in the ancient traditions is more than just heat. It also represents *light,* and it helps us to see. Through the subtle fields the liver is connected to the eyes, and they often give a first indication that the fire is aggravated and burning too high (the eyes become reddened), or if it is weak from being overworked or the overwork has led to the beginning of a disease process (the whites of the eyes may take on a yellow hue if the bilirubin is out of balance). Subtler yet, a balanced inner fire helps the mind to perceive clearly; it ignites our intellect so it can better understand ideas, "digest" concepts, and assimilate positive thoughts while discarding negative ones. The yogi refers to this clarity as giving us the capacity for "right thinking," the ability to perceive the truth of the situation before you.

Given this connection, it is no surprise that the liver is the organ most connected to our mental body, the subtle field of energy that holds how we perceive not only ourselves but also the world around us. Our mind is our gateway to our higher nature—when the mind becomes still, we can step beyond thought to experience the oneness of our being—and the liver "lights the way" to connect with our higher desire to seek oneness.

In clinical practice, when the liver is in balance, supported, and not overworked, our perception is more clear, our thinking is more sharp, and our outlook is positive. When it is not, the heat of too much fire building up disturbs the balance of the elements: The heating of water and air creates a fog of hot steam that obfuscates our vision. In this state, we might make assumptions and misjudgments or become "fired up" about how right we are, causing confrontations in our relationships. We might become convinced of a truth that is actually just a mirage. If the liver function gets congested, the fire of the liver can build up in intensity and express as irritation, frustration, or anger—or get repressed as simmering and unspoken resentment. And vice versa: If we frequently erupt in anger, our blood heats up and creates inflammation, as well as anger, that the liver must then process.

The process of health always involves tending to the fire through awareness of diet, of our fluctuations in positive and negative mind-set, and of the effect of rising stress levels, so as to ensure it neither blazes out of control nor falls too low, damp and dim. Some people naturally have more fire or *pitta dosha* in their body type, and for them excessive fire comes easily, so they learn to temper the diet of spicy foods and use the breath to cool the heat in times of aggravation. For other types, disharmony in the liver creates a deficiency and weakness in the fire element. Both can be brought to balance so that metabolism, mind-set, digestion, and skin are better.

I understand the fire in the solar plexus chakra through an additional dimension: A well-balanced fire unlocks the etheric energy imbued in good food, helping it on its path from the earth's field to that of our body. In chapter 1 you learned that etheric energy *comes into* the physical body through the endocrine glands; in the solar plexus chakra, the pancreas is the corresponding endocrine gland and the liver communicates with the pancreas, existing in close relationship with it. Through the digestion of good food that is imbued with electromagnetic energy, the energy of the food is absorbed and nourishes our own electromagnetic field. *This* is one of the reasons we want to eat good organic food and also carefully stoke this digestive flame, through cleansing the liver of congestion and stress and cooking and combining foods properly, as you will learn to do in Part Two. From the sacred fire emerges the mantra that I share with every patient in order to remind them to live a lifestyle of loving their liver, their lymph, and their powerful digestive force: *What you eat matters; how your body processes what you eat matters even more!*

## THE LYMPH SYSTEM

Over the decades that I worked in the Sri Lankan free clinic with Professor Anton, we taught patients the power of nature's least expensive medicine: conscious breathing. We did this because it helps to move the lymph fluid through the intricate system of tubes, glands (including the spleen and tonsils), and nodes that compose the lymphatic system—a rarely mentioned second circulatory system in the body that draws out waste and impurities from our tissues and carries them into the bloodstream to be taken to the liver and kidneys for processing and elimination. The lymph system helps to cleanse the tissues of the brain of accumulated proteins and waste to support cognitive function. Much of the lymph fluid in the system is produced in the liver from plasma filtered out of the blood as it passes through the lymph system and organ tissues.

The lymph system is like the drainage system of the body, helping unwanted materials and excess fluids move downstream toward the exit instead of accumulating in our tissues. It maintains the correct fluid balance in the body, and when it's clear and working well, we might appreciate that our skin looks hydrated and smooth and not puffy or bumpy. It is also an essential part of our immune system: When the spleen and lymph nodes receive information that an invading parasite has been identified—typically alerted by the lymphatic tissue that lines the outside of the intestinal wall and scans for the presence of foreign materials—they produce white blood cells, which enter the bloodstream and defend the body against these organisms. If the lymph is congested, this essential immune function gets hampered and we get sick more often. The lymph has a third powerful duty: It transports fatty acids to the liver to get burned as fuel. Unlike most dissolved nutrients, which go from the intestine straight into the bloodstream, fatty acids take a lap in the lymph fluid first. Healthy lymph is therefore key if we want to enjoy sustained energy; when the lymphatic circulation is stagnant, it hinders healthy fat metabolism and we can feel especially tired.

Despite all these extraordinary endeavors, the lymph system gets even less attention than the liver in modern Western medicine—it is unseen and underappreciated for all its efforts in helping us to feel energized and resilient. Fortunately, many of the steps that take care of the liver also take care of the lymph system, as you will learn in Part Two (with a few special extra techniques to bring into your lifestyle). Unlike the blood, which is pumped around its circulatory system by the heart, the circulation of the lymph has to be encouraged through our mechanical movements, like good breaths that expand and contract the rib cage, as well as movement of the whole body—be it through yoga asanas, walking, running, dancing, swimming, or bouncing. Lymphatic circulation also benefits from dry skin brushing, which is outlined on page 180. If you've barely considered your lymph system before, you will come to appreciate why loving your lymph goes hand in hand with loving your liver.

## The Liver in Esoteric Understanding: The "Filter"

The third aspect of the liver is the most esoteric, and it has to do with the etheric nature of the blood. If you have ever wondered why in many cultures the blood is considered to be the symbol of life, it is not merely because this fluid contains the red blood cells that carry oxygen and the white blood cells that fight infection. The blood is a powerful resonator of etheric energy, in much the same way that water conducts electricity. It is an extraordinary carrier of the etheric energy that flows through our subtle anatomy and enlivens our physical self.

The liver filters and purifies the blood: Physically it filters all the blood in the body from contaminants, and etherically it purifies and tonifies the blood of emotional and mental toxins in order to promote a flow in the etheric body. Emotions and thoughts can have biochemical responses in the body and are frequencies that can either resonate with our etheric body or, depending on the nature of the emotion, interfere with it. Uplifting and expansive emotions like joy and love do the former; difficult or contracting emotions like grief and anger do the latter.

Nature designed our emotional and mental responses to be fleeting; they are momentary reactions to stimuli that occur in order to catalyze us into an action. When in fear, we move to safety in order to survive; when in anger, we can make a good choice (or what yogis sometimes know as "right action") to correct an injustice, and when in joy and love, we connect and share to experience serenity and contentment. Positive emotions are healing to the liver. We know that from the way our mood surges or heart flutters when we have them. Joy, happiness, and love pass through us like butterflies on the wind or shooting stars across the sky. Challenging emotions like fear, anger, resentment, rage, anxiety, and envy, however, have a low vibration; after the initial rush of emotion or surge of injustice we might feel, they do not dissolve quite as effortlessly. To put it another way, they have a tendency to block the liver's energy, causing fatigue and exhaustion. The liver is the organ that filters these emotional and mental frequencies through the blood. When we repress emotions rather than acknowledge them, this can lead to stagnation. If the liver is working well and our mental outlook has clarity, then we can "let go" of challenging emotions and we can gain awareness of how to live in harmony with ourselves.

Understanding the liver's filtering capacity in a multidimensional way helps us to appreciate the significance of cleansing the liver. A program to keep the liver at optimal function becomes more than an annual detox; it becomes part of a lifestyle of enjoying clarity and connection. When the liver can detoxify the toxins in the blood, the etheric energy is free to resonate coherently. We radiate with energy, we feel supported by our reserves, and our etheric energy moves harmoniously between our physical and subtle fields, helping us to feel more in touch with ourselves and with nature. By caring for one of our important organs, the liver, we can begin to live with a greater state of awareness.

## SATTVA, RAJAS, TAMAS: THE BALANCE OF THREE

From an Ayurvedic perspective, we see that in order for the blood to best resonate etheric energy, it must be in balance with its triune (threefold) nature. The element of "purity" or *sattva* is important for this balance, for *sattva* is the neutral *guna*, or the universal force of consciousness, that we experience as purity in thoughts, words, and actions. In our modern, high-stress world, *sattva* must balance the two other *gunas*: *rajas*—the energy of stimulation and excitement—and *tamas*, the energy of laziness and inertia. Today most of us are influenced by this polarized play of *rajas* and *tamas*—hyperactivity that can manifest in the form of addictions on one end and lack of interest in yourself and the world around you on the other end.

From a subtle medicine point of view, we may see the two poles as the electric and the magnetic fields. Ayurveda teaches that the liver's job is to help clear the blood of excess *tamas* and *rajas* in order for them to be in balance with *sattva*. It is the universal law of the balance of threes (the triune function): *Sattvic* purity is balanced with *tamas* to relax and enjoy the flow but not to become stagnant, and *rajas* to move forward in action, but without the "go, go, go" of the modern world.

# The Force of the Mental Will

Have you ever noticed that when you are sick and run down, everyday tasks feel pointless and larger life goals seem utterly out of reach? Your fire for life has dwindled and your desire to take care of things in your world—and participate in the world at large—dwindles with it. This is a clue that your connection to your will is getting weak . . . and without your will, it is hard to be well. In Harmonic Healing the will is a supersubtle aspect of our vitality that supports our vital force, enabling us to heal.

Rising out of the fire of the liver and reverberating through the mental body, the mental will is the energy that drives us forward with determination and conviction. It is the force that wills us to carry on to something more, even when challenges are in our path. The will is the strongest aspect of the healing potential. Here's why: Action, intention, and purpose connect our physical body to our higher nature.

The action comes from our *physical will* to be, which resides in the base chakra, where the adrenals have the capacity to generate energy under stressful conditions for the fight-or-flight response. The intention comes from our *mental will* to be, which resides in the solar plexus chakra, where the liver processes our thoughts. It is the self-awareness and the desire behind the statement *"I will."* The purpose of our *spiritual will* to be, resides in the crown chakra and resonates with the ajna chakra and inspires us to see, and to put intention into action, by connecting us to our purpose. The power of intention comes from our mental and spiritual bodies resonating with each other and connects our purpose and action.

I have found that it is important to have a strong mental will to sustain health. While many are aware that supporting our detoxification organs is important, few realize that this is one of the central reasons why. As beings of free will, we have a choice in everything we do; we have a choice to make one small positive step in difficult times, a choice to pick the healing food or the junk food, a choice to breathe a full breath or to shut down and tighten up. With our mental will, we decide to make those better choices. One might equate the mental will to belief, and in some ways it is. But the mental will is more than belief; it is a thread of consciousness that ripples through the subtle fields and connects the physical to the subtle communication. The mental will is the secret behind the power of the mind to heal. Simply stated, the force of the solar plexus, the radiating sun, directs our life.

A patient may say, "I am feeling better!" even if they still have more layers to clear on their health journey. The "I am" in the statement "I am feeling better" is always a sign that the mental will is back.. This can look many ways—either a deeper commitment to a path of spiritual practice they are already on or simply a few moments in the day of pausing from the mundane to acknowledge and be grateful for nature or a connection to others. The liver, our hardworking factory, is a connection to our higher purpose.

## What the Liver Needs to Do Its Work

Given the extraordinary range of work that the liver performs, what does this star organ of the digestive force, glowing radiantly in the very energy center of our body, need in order to do its best?

You will discover the ideal conditions as you read through Part Two. Here's a preview: Your kitchen would be filled with a bounty of fresh and seasonal fruits and vegetables that support digestion and detoxification, from beets to apples to sulfur-containing vegetables like broccoli, cauliflower, and cabbage (detoxification requires the mineral sulfur to be in our diet). You might also infuse your food with spices like turmeric that support liver cell regeneration and combat inflammation, and you'd eat them calmly and intentionally, in simple combinations, with natural and unprocessed fats as your staples. You would turn off your devices during meals knowing that too much visual and mental stimulation interferes with good digestion. You would drink clean water in a natural way to support the flow of bile and lymph and would relax into your breathing as you worked, played, and rested. Furthermore, you wouldn't stay seated for the whole day—you would move often so that your lymph stayed fluidly mobile too. If any minor aches or pains occurred, you would find a remedy from nature, sidestepping nonessential pharmaceutical drugs that can aggravate the liver and disrupt normal functioning. You'd finish eating several hours before bedtime, take some moments to unwind at the end of the day and release any unresolved emotions (such as with the Ho'oponopono prayer of forgiveness), and fall easily and happily asleep for several hours before the 1:00 A.M. window when the fire or *pitta* in our body naturally rises and encourages the liver to do its cleansing work.

Now ask yourself, how many of these ideal experiences are constants in your everyday life? A few of these things may already be daily occurrences; or perhaps none of them occur regularly for you. Instead of all these things being aspects of our everyday reality, they are more like glaring lacks. This means that our liver and our digestive force all too often suffer from a dearth of the ingredients and support they require. In fact, they typically get handed quite the opposite.

## And What the Liver Gets: The Congesting and Inflammatory Effects of Modern Life

Even before we make any of our everyday lifestyle choices, the invisible effects of our modern milieu are at work. The fields of pollution create interference with the cells' energy patterns, weakening the function of the liver, gallbladder, and pancreas and creating inflammation throughout our body. The stomach, on the other hand, is also part of the solar plexus chakra and is where heavy metals can suppress hydrochloric acid, hindering the first step of protein digestion. If the stomach cannot properly process proteins, then another burden of digestion is on the liver.

Into this already weakened environment enters an extraordinary additional set of digestive and detoxification demands. The plethora includes processed foods, factory-farmed foods, extremely high levels of sugars that stress the pancreas and the liver in tandem as they synthesize and store the glucose, prescription medications, excessive amounts of stimulating caffeine and alcohol (which require effortful metabolizing), and the greatest hazard to the liver and gallbladder of all: unnatural fats.

## Fats Matter

From the liver's point of view, the twentieth-century shift to refined plant oils like canola oil, corn oil, soybean oil, and the falsely named "vegetable oil" (which doesn't contain any vegetables) can be the straw that breaks the camel's back. These fats are pervasive, used in processed foods, restaurants, fast-food chains, and very often the kitchen at home. Where minimally processed oils like extra-virgin olive oil are fairly effortlessly emulsified by the bile and broken down into fatty acids before crossing into the lymph system and then the bloodstream, the molecular structure of *refined* oils has been damaged by processing and is then typically further damaged by cooking at high heat. The fat molecules become jagged instead of remaining round and smooth, which has an inflammatory and congesting effect instead of the healing effect of unheated olive oil on the liver. I have come to observe how this damage happens by heating oils on high heat—except grape-seed oil, ghee, and the naturally occurring fat in meats. The protective antidotes to this include simple dietary habits, such as using unheated extra-virgin olive oil as a condiment for our fat needs in our diet and learning to cook without using oils on high heat, instead employing a low and slow cooking method that can even be done without any cooked oils to help cleanse the liver and give it a rest from the inflammation that can be caused by heated oils. We will explore this in Part Two.

Though the focus on minimally heated fats may seem like a side note, it is all-important. It is difficult for the liver to process fat molecules damaged from high heat. And it is healing for the liver to digest unheated raw virgin olive oil in its natural state. Unemulsified fats can sit in the intestines awaiting digestion and can begin to congest the shared duct that brings bile and enzymes from their sources (the gallbladder and the pancreas) into the intestines. This can cause the digestion to weaken, because the bile and the pancreatic juices together perform the majority of the digestive effort. Without their normal passage into the small intestine, we may begin to experience bloating, digestive distress after eating, and lack of motility in the intestines, which can lead into constipation. Undigested fats that accumulate in the blood can cause the blood to become heavy and laden with fats, causing stress on circulation and the heart. Very often high blood pressure is caused by the heart having to push around this heavy, fatty blood.

Because bile also helps to buffer any hydrochloric acid that overflows from the stomach into the first part of the small intestine, a slowdown in bile triggers the body to turn *down* the normal acid production in the stomach, weakening digestion further still. One result can be that harder-to-digest foods that never caused a problem before, like gluten and dairy, begin to create digestive distress. This can lead us to eliminate those food groups entirely in an effort to solve the distress, which may temporarily alleviate symptoms but does not necessarily get to the root cause: a weakened liver and congested ducts asking to be cleansed!

If liver congestion goes on for too long, other issues can arise. Gallstones can form from an excess of bile that builds up in a sluggish gallbladder. When they accumulate, they can inhibit the free flow of bile, further inhibiting digestion, and can lodge in the bile and pancreatic ducts, causing inflammation that may require medical attention. Furthermore, congested blood in the portal system of the liver—the circulatory system that brings blood from the intestines to the liver—can be the cause of hemorrhoids, due to the impact on the hemorrhoidal vein at the end of the portal system.

## Intensifying the Effect

It's not *just* about the oils we select. Our carbohydrate consumption can burden the liver further if we fall into poor patterns. The liver metabolizes all carbohydrates and stores the extra as glycogen. A relatively recent phenomenon has drastically intensified the liver's workload: the high levels of fructose in our modern diets, which far exceed what we evolved to consume, thanks to the proliferation of sucrose and the overuse of fructose sweetening in processed foods and drinks. When consumption exceeds the small amounts we evolved to eat from seasonal fruits, the liver can get overloaded and will convert the fructose to fat. If this accumulates, the fat in the liver can initiate metabolic chaos and insulin resistance and lead to conditions like obesity and diabetes, so prevalent today. This is why as part of caring for the liver and its sister organ, the pancreas, we want to take good care to remove all artificial fructose-containing products from the diet and be conscious of our use of excess sugar. Even honey, which confers many wonderful protective benefits when unheated, needs to be served with a very judicious hand.

At the other extreme, withholding proper nutrition by being excessively stringent with carbohydrate consumption, such as by following an extreme low-carb diet or restricting calories in general for too long, can cause its own kind of strain. Glycogen stores can run too low, and if we are not digesting fats well enough to burn them for fuel instead—a metabolic state that requires intentional effort and consistency in diet to achieve—the body is forced to use an emergency energy source, the stress hormones created by the adrenals, in a desperate attempt to "power on" in life. If this becomes a pattern, it can weaken the adrenals and then the thyroid, contributing to systemic exhaustion.

To those who have adopted a very low-carbohydrate diet filled with high-caloric fats either to avoid grains that are irritating their systems or to replace starches that are destabilizing blood sugar, I invite a reframing. We need fats as fuel for warmth; they also support our well-being because they have a soothing and pacifying effect. Yet they can confer these benefits only if we can digest them well and absorb them into our blood. When high quantities of fats are consumed by a body that is struggling to digest them, we are facilitating the congested conditions described in this chapter, which can slowly accumulate without our realizing it.

Rather than replacing all grains and all starchy carbohydrates in the diet with higher levels of fat in order to try to resolve weight and blood-sugar issues, I often suggest an alternative route in order to avoid the risks of liver congestion. I typically have the patient *restore the digestive force first* by following the Liver-Cleansing Diet, focusing on improving their relationship with vegetables first and foremost and enjoying moderate amounts of good fats, rather than adding copious amounts of extra fats.

Clearing a congested liver and loosening the grip of a parasite such as candida can often be the two keys that shift the original symptoms of weight and inflammation, allowing the body to digest organic whole grains. This approach helps to create a lifestyle replete with a broader array of foods that includes complex carbohydrates—with the addition of easy-to-assimilate good unheated fats to support our nervous system. There are exceptions to this rule; for instance, those whose bodies have a tendency toward blood-sugar issues will do better staying off grains and starches for a period of time while increasing protein as the blood sugar begins to normalize. But very often the person who has diligently avoided gluten for years may find that a whole-grain pasta made with organic grains can be nurturing and rebuilding for the body when the liver is ready to metabolize the carbohydrate.

## Liver Overload: The Ripple Effect

If the digestive force gets weakened, all kinds of imbalances can ensue. The buildup of mucus from poorly digested proteins can trap parasites and their larvae in the mucus lining of the intestinal tract and we can become bloated, puffier, and more tired and feel more uncomfortable in our body. One reason for this is that the delicate lymphatic tissue in the intestinal wall is a "border crossing" through which fatty acids—in an unusual anomaly of the digestive process—get absorbed into the lymph system before being moved into the bloodstream. When the lacteal tissue becomes congested by the presence of undigested fats, bloating or stubborn weight around our midsection is a common result.

As the poorly emulsified fats make their way into the lymph fluid, they cause congestion in the lymphatic circulation. This can allow toxins to accumulate in the tissues and inhibit the circulation of immune cells to where they are needed in times of infection or injury. When this occurs, we might feel more aches and pains, experience swelling or puffiness in the face and all over our body, or discover cellulite from the congesting fat that causes changes in the skin's texture. We might experience hardening in the breasts from congestion in the breasts' lymphatic tissue; or as the major glands of the lymphatic system—the thymus, tonsils, and spleen—become weakened, we might start getting sick more often or become more vulnerable to opportunistic parasites.

The lymphatic congestion is exacerbated by sedentary behavior and the constricted breathing that becomes normal when stress and busyness dominate. When the lymphatic function diminishes, even more pressure is put on the liver to detoxify. Combine this with the habit of late nights that disrupt the natural cleansing cycles of the liver, plus the bombardment of information that tends to keep us in a state of hypervigilance unless we actively take steps to change it, and no wonder the absorption of the energy and nutrients from food is low and we have moments of exhaustion as a result.

**OH, NUTS!**

Nuts (and nut milks, flours, and butters) are often used to replace grains and dairy, but consuming nuts in large amounts comes with side effects. Because of their concentrated fat and protein content, nuts can be hard to digest. On the Liver-Cleansing Diet, nuts are removed from the diet to allow the liver to rest from this concentrated harder-to-digest protein and reintroduced later in moderate amounts. Today nut consumption can really creep up on us without our realizing how much we are consuming. Nuts should not be eaten as we eat popcorn at a movie but used as the concentrated protein they are and eaten according to the food-combining rules. Nuts and nut butters can be used in small quantities.

## Toxic Accumulation and Disharmony in the Liver

As the liver tries to keep up with life's unrelenting demands, it can quite easily fall into disharmony, and the detoxification processes can get overwhelmed. Our blood needs to be cleansed of physical and emotional and mental toxins in an ongoing fashion; when the wave of incoming toxins becomes a tsunami, many are left unprocessed, and this can make the blood inflamed. We can experience this inflammation as heat in different parts of the body, causing seemingly non-liver-related issues like arthritis; high blood pressure; problematic skin reactions like acne, rosacea, or boils; migraine headaches and pressure at the temples and around the eyes; nausea; muscle tightness and pain in the shoulders; sciatica; and hot flashes. As with every extreme, the reverse can also occur. If our personal tendency is to lose our "fire" or *pitta* when under stress, an overwhelmed liver can leave us looking ashy and dulled, as if the fire has dwindled too low.

Disharmony in the liver can also lead to weight gain. Our bodies want to keep us protected from the unprocessed, fat-soluble toxins that, due to liver stagnation, have not been converted to water-soluble toxins that can be excreted. To take these toxins out of circulation, it parks them safely away in the fat cells, including the fat cells in the brain or around the organs or glands; its innate intelligence is to keep the fat so that the toxins don't start to circulate. Quite often, the body resists all attempts to lose the extra weight through dieting and exercise—at least until the liver is cleansed enough and relieved of stress and can handle the load of toxins that will be released.

The accumulation in the blood of used-up hormones, which have been left unprocessed by a tired liver, also contributes to stubborn pounds, compounding the situation. Depending on which hormone dominates, the distribution of the excess weight can lead to a pear shape or apple shape of the body. Hormone imbalance of the estrogen hormone can meanwhile cause changes in overall reproductive health.

The ripple effect of accumulated toxins can spread to many places; toxins can accumulate in the neurological system of nerves and the brain. Because the liver/solar plexus chakra is connected to the heart chakra through the etheric field, an overly stressed liver often expresses in the heart, manifesting as symptoms like high blood pressure, circulatory issues, clogged arteries, or an "angry heart." The congestion and inflammation initiated in the liver ripples through the subtle bodies, and this is when we start to have trouble digesting our lives. We may find ourselves responding to circumstances by being irritable, angry, or resentful, with volatile surges of temper. Depending on our temperament and constitution, we may find ourselves more stuck than enraged—stuck in our mental outlook, stubborn, hardened to others—and find it difficult to feel or empathize. This blocked energy brings down our outlook and mood, turning it dark, negative, and depressed. The word *melancholy* comes from the Greek *melancholia,* which translates to "black bile," and from the earliest days of medicine, stagnant bile and liver function was seen as a root of depression and malaise. Interestingly, the word *bile* itself is defined as ill temper and peevishness, and the definition of *gall* is bitterness of spirit and rancor. Anyone familiar with Shakespeare has heard the bard's protagonists proclaim, "The gall of him!" Our language points to what occurs when these parts of ourselves are allowed to become extreme.

And when, as described above, the overwhelmed liver struggles to clear negative emotions from the blood, these unhelpful feelings and mental states can stay in circulation. We might continue to feel them as reverberations and as feelings we can't let go, though we may not be conscious of why. Over time, these challenging emotional feelings and mental thoughts can become part of our temperament and become part of our story about "who we are." Should this occur, it can be helpful to find someone who will listen to your story, whether it is a therapist, a family member, or a trusted friend—being heard can help us to gain self-awareness—or even do a course of nonviolent communication, which is another way to help bring peace to our feelings and thoughts and to learn deep listening. We want to take the necessary steps to let go of negative thoughts and emotions before they become crystallized matter that can even lead to physical changes. For example, bile can harden from crystallized angry thoughts to form gallstones in the liver and gallbladder and can be difficult to release, while blocking our fat digestion.

If the liver is weak, the will of the mental body can be weak. We can feel defeated or trapped in inertia, unable to motivate or to stick to our decisions. In this state, the decision to eat well, live well, and love ourselves is harder to make. In Harmonic Healing we understand that congestion and blocks can occur in the physical body and in the subtle fields; when the etheric energy of the liver is suppressed, we can even lose our connection to our divine nature, that which connects our mental understanding to our knowing of our purpose and our place in the world.

It is no surprise that in many cases of illness the overburdened liver is involved. Supporting the body's healing and rejuvenation potential starts with cleansing the liver and supplying our body with organic, energy-rich whole food.

Fran came to me when she was in her forties, after a full profile of blood tests failed to give clues as to why her usual high energy had dropped and she felt older and more tired than she suspected was normal at her age. The blood tests had all been in the normal range, and her doctor said there was nothing he could recommend to improve her health. Yet Fran knew she was functioning and thinking more slowly than she had in her twenties and thirties. She didn't believe that being in her forties was a valid reason for feeling this way.

My evaluation showed a high level of toxins in the blood and poorly functioning organs of digestion, even though these findings had not been revealed through the standard blood tests for high lipids or elevated liver enzymes. Or at least, not yet! I told her that by working at the prephysical level we can become aware of imbalances early and make changes before the imbalance manifests as the first stages of disease.

Excited to have her instincts validated, Fran followed the Liver-Cleansing Program and then transitioned into a lifestyle of caring for her liver. Her vitality returned and she told me that she felt as vibrant as an eight-year-old, and she noticed how the clearer her body became, the clearer her perception became too. She reported "a truly earth-shattering moment" driving on the interstate. Completely unflustered by other drivers cutting her off or speeding past her aggressively, she felt "like all my inner edges were smoothed" and as if she'd found a place of inner calmness and contentment she hadn't known before. She saw how this state reverberated from her newly "happy liver" at her center. Now almost sixty and a longtime follower of the lifestyle, Fran reports that her vitality remains high, her body feels great, her mind is clear and sharp, and her emotions calm and content. She has gained mastery over her own health.

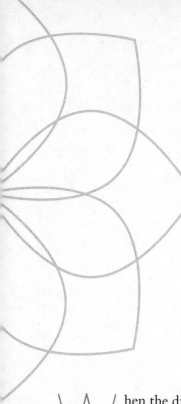

Chapter 5

# Conscious Nutrition: The Sacred Power of Food

When the digestive fire—the sun at our solar plexus chakra—is burning bright and strong, it lights the way of health through the digestive process and assimilation of food that nourishes our life force.

We absorb the subtle energies of nature and the cosmos through many channels—from the air we breathe, the sun's rays, and the earth's electromagnetic field. While we can learn practices that harness the subtle energy of air and sun, and even harness the earth's energy in subtle ways such as walking barefoot, first things first. In health we start from the ground up, and when it comes to nourishing our etheric energy, we start with what we eat.

New patients who arrive at the clinic are very often subsisting on energetically depleted foods. This scenario never surprises, for we are living in an era of depletion, and nowhere does the phenomenon hit harder than in the nutritional quality of our food. Yet while collectively we're beginning to wake up to some of the missing pieces in nutrition, our attention tends to land on the obvious issues of concern: portion sizes, refined grains, excess sugar, processed foods, and rancid fats.

Seeing food as more than physical sustenance and as the very source of life is not as mysterious as it may seem. We have always been connected to the subtle power of food; we have traditionally revered the edible plants we harvest and the creatures of land or sea that give us nourishment. We perform rituals as we sow seeds, pray for rain, and process crops; we bless food as we prepare it in the kitchen, and we give gratitude for nature before enjoying the meal. This gratitude for the life-giving energy that causes seeds to sprout, shoots to grow, and fruit to ripen, and that also helps our cells to respire and our brains to cognize, came from an understanding that the growing forces of nature exist in harmony with the healing forces of our body, and nature, if left to her own devices, will give us what we need. But in the rush of progress and our shift to convenience, the consciousness of food's subtle, sacred nature has gotten lost.

A conscious connection to eating can look many ways, but the simplest is this: choosing to fill our plates and bowls with simple, fresh, whole food ingredients from good sources, combined with care and eaten with pleasure. When this habit becomes installed, it is a pillar of health that supports us to let go of overly restrictive diets and cease chasing the next fad food program, and dispels the anxiety around what we eat. Food imbued with etheric life energy restores and regenerates.

## The Subtle Nature of Food

The ancient ways teach us that food is more than a source of sustenance; it is the foundation of health. One of the earliest medical doctrines, written by the Indian scholar Sushruta Samhita, notes, "By changing dietary habits the human organism may be cured without using any medicine, while with hundreds of good medicines, diseases of the human organism cannot be cured if the food is wrong. Right food is the only key to good health."

Both Ayurveda and Chinese medicine arose from concepts of how energy moves inside us and in relationship with our environment. They consider a properly chosen diet to be the first line of treatment for well-being, prescribed even before an herbal tincture or therapeutic tea is given or a hands-on treatment is applied. The knowledge of these early subtle medicines, handed down in the kitchen and shared in the doctor's clinic, teaches that the right food is a fundamental tool for creating conditions in the body that resist disease and encourage longevity.

Subtle medicines approach diet in a slightly different way from the way we do today. Where the modern Western paradigm is predominantly concerned with quantity—how much food to ingest and how many calories this delivers—in subtle medicines the primary focus is on the energy of the food and the actions these initiate in the body after it's consumed. Rather than categorizing foods as "good" or "bad," subtler approaches see all healthfully cultivated food as having inherent health-giving properties. It is a *relational* understanding of food that looks at the food *and* the person consuming it; it acknowledges how our individual tendencies influence the ways we digest foods and metabolize them for fuel, and whether we burn our fuel efficiently or store it on our body as fat. Unlike the exclusive approach of the rigid diets and programs that have come to the forefront of the wellness industry today, the subtler approach is inclusive. It uses the bounty of nature's offerings, both from the plant world—the roots and tubers that grow underground, the leaves and fronds that sprout from the soil, and the fruits that reach to the sky—and from the animal world.

In this approach, the tastes or flavors of a food, the density and texture of it, and, very important, its heating or cooling properties are considered decisive factors in how "healthy" it may be for one person versus another. All these properties have the potential to affect the functioning of our organs, glands, and systems, as well as our state of mind and emotions, because they affect the balance of air, fire, and water within us—the three elements or energies of nature that underlie our individual makeups and that govern our physical and mental processes. Furthermore, the subtle paradigm takes into consideration our bodies' fluctuating responses to seasonal, climatic, or even circumstantial changes in our lives. In plainest terms, nutrition is more than physical; it is multidimensional. And through cultivating a very basic awareness, such as noticing the sensation of becoming overheated or chilled as the seasons change or detecting anxious or ungrounded feelings in different phases of our lives, we can choose foods to address imbalances early, before they become symptoms that lead into disease.

In the early years of working with patients, first as a chef in the yoga ashram restaurant and subsequently through nutritional counseling, this knowledge of the subtle power of food became the foundation of a healing philosophy based on the medicinal properties of plants, spices, and herbs; whole grains and legumes and good sources of protein and fats; and low and slow methods of cooking.

At the foundation of nutrition is food in its original whole form; grown in healthy, chemical-free soil, minimally processed using gentle cooking methods, and free of packaging. As I worked with patients to restore their vitality and witnessed the transforming effects of a diverse, fresh, whole-foods diet, it became clear that the healing potential of food was intrinsically linked to something even finer and more discreet than the tastes, textures, and temperature properties. It came down to the electromagnetic energy in foods grown the way nature intended.

## Discovering the Unseen Energy of Food

You have learned that the vehicle in which you live is a *physical-etheric* body composed of physical matter that supports, carries, and holds you and a subtle field of etheric energy that radiates through and around you, feeding into the physical to enliven it with vitality.

And so it is with food.

In Chinese philosophy, the symbol for the unseen etheric energy—known as qi (also spelled chi or ki)—is a grain of rice cooking. Rice in Asian cultures is an extremely important ingredient for nutrition. The symbol illustrates not only the solid, nutritive grain of rice but also the transformation that takes place when the rice is boiled or steamed. The rice grain changes from a hard kernel of potential energy to an easily digested fuel. Qi is the substance of the grain, the energy needed to transform the grain, and the steam vapor that occurs when cooking. Qi is both substantial and ephemeral, seen and unseen, form and formless, static and movable. To understand how plants are imbued with this subtle energy, let's put our attention on a realm of nature that is often over-looked: the mineral kingdom.

## The Magic of Minerals

The soil, the plants, and the animal kingdom need a constant supply of minerals to sustain life and growth. Trace minerals are tiny, but they carry the force that builds new tissue and maintains general health and are catalytic in action. These mineral constituents are found in our blood and in every cell of our body. Rare trace minerals are catalysts that function throughout our system and form the action that promotes our enzyme activity that is required for health.

It is fairly well established that minerals are essential for physiological functions in the body to occur—iron carries oxygen in the blood, sulfur helps the detoxification pathways, and calcium creates bones and teeth—and when we are depleted of minerals, many of these functions suffer, and we get increasingly tired. But they play an important, often overlooked, subtle purpose. Our life force especially utilizes the trace elements from our food. Minerals emanate an electromagnetic field, in a similar way to crystals used in energy healing for their ability to emanate different frequencies. Minerals hold the electromagnetic energy of the earth's field.

Although the word "mineral" may make you think of hard, inert substances, it is important to recognize that plants, which can be leafy, delicate, and distinctly non-rock-like, are also part of the mineral kingdom. Minerals from the earth's soil dissolve in water to form mineral salts which are especially abundant around the roots—particularly if the soil is organic and not depleted by chemical inputs. I find that the quantity and quality of these minute nutrients are highest in vegetable foods, over grains and legumes. Plants use these substances along with the water from the soil and the light of the sun as catalysts of their own life activity, helping them to germinate from seed, emerge from the soil, and grow. And if that's not magic enough, here is where it gets even better: As the plants take up the mineral salts through the roots, the mineral-filled plants emanate electromagnetic energy. When we eat and digest these plants, our bodies resonate with and absorb electromagnetic energy for our etheric field. Because they act as the energetic bridge between the earth's electromagnetic energy field and our body's energy field, I consider plants to be our most important connection to Mother Earth's healing potential.

## Soil: Our Source of Life

Years of close work with Dr. Hazel Parcells led me to a deeper understanding about our modern-day, depleted foods. Her understanding of the energy of food was extraordinary, and it helped to reveal *why* the quality of food we eat matters so much. Using the tools of radiesthesia, which can detect and quantify the electromagnetic energy emanating from anything with a life force, we measured the fields of energy of countless foods and evaluated them. It became clear that while all food has the *potential* to have electromagnetic energy, this energy is more present if the source of the food is free of heavy metals, pesticides, and petrochemicals.

Unfortunately, much of the world's soil has been severely depleted by agricultural processes, such as monocropping and overfarming, that do not allow soil to recover the rich mix of minerals between growing seasons. Agricultural processes like these, though born of good intentions to feed rapidly expanding populations, take and take but do not restore and replenish the soil through rotational cover crops, the way farmers always used to. As a result of decades of this kind of treatment, the depletion level of soil has reached a disturbing extreme. In direct reflection of this, most conventionally grown foods have a low electromagnetic field. The fact that many foods are picked early, before natural ripening occurs, then transported long distances before sale, further diminishes their energy. Another modern practice, that of forcing produce to unnaturally large sizes, has made sugar content in the fruits and vegetables higher but minerals lower; this supersize, supermarket-friendly produce often has lower energetic potential and a low concentration of nutrients.

Foods cultivated in depleted soils may sustain us, and we can live on them, but these foods are low in minerals that support electromagnetic energy, and do not feed our etheric field, our reserve energy; a Chinese-medicine practitioner would say they are deficient in qi. When they are our primary source of nutrition, illness and digestive disturbances can appear.

On top of this fundamental depletion, toxic substances, which are present in chemical fertilizers, pesticides, herbicides, and fungicides, create a low electromagnetic field. Further, chemical additives are used in multiple steps of processing, from harvesting to ripening to displaying to processing into packaged goods, and there is interference from the packaging materials themselves. Not surprisingly, when foods grown with or laden with chemicals are eaten every day, they interfere with *our* electromagnetic field and bring our vitality down. Foods that are radiated for sanitization, such as spices, have no vibrational frequency at all; they are virtually "dead" and will also bring down our electromagnetic energy. (Interestingly, homeopathic remedies can lose their potency when they are passed through the airport scanners during travel, which is why these items should not go through security checkpoints unless in a lead X-ray film bag—and why we may want to opt out of the airport security scanners as well.)

In the 1970s and 1980s, when I researched the energetics of food, it was not easy to explain the phenomenon to most. The alternative to conventionally produced food, organic food, was the outlier at this time—a small niche market for back-to-nature types. Some voices contended, as they still do today, that the nutritional potential of conventional and organic foods is comparable. Yet the clinical results could not be denied. Over and again, evaluations showed that the cellular balance of those who ate organically grown food free of chemical interference, and whose digestive system was working well, enjoyed energy in the cells and thus a healthy and restored vital force. They were more resilient to stress and better able to withstand the interferences of our modern world. Their food was not only giving their organs and tissues the required nutrients; it was feeding their etheric body.

Going beyond organic food, we found that biodynamic food was even more energetically potent. Biodynamic food is grown in ways that intentionally harness the subtle energetic forces of the cosmos, for example by planting and harvesting in sync with the lunar cycle. Wild foods such as berries, greens, herbs, and roots foraged in nature have similarly enhanced potential because they have grown in environments that have been untouched by man's hand, and they are naturally growing in harmony with the seasons and rhythms of the earth. The fact that a new market of wild-crafted foods and biodynamic products is establishing itself in today's era speaks volumes about this—those who use them appreciate the heightened vitality they get from food that is so directly connected to source.

We found that the energy of the food has its highest potential right after picking, because the growing forces are still present; they diminish in energy as the plant ages. And young foods like sprouts have high nutritional potential because they are filled with the growing forces of nature; sprouts are the plant bursting out from seed and into life. But it's not just vegetables, fruits, and herbs that contain etheric energy. In plant proteins like lentils and legumes, as well as grains, if the food is cultivated chemically free, a high potential will likely be measured. The same goes for toxin-free animal-derived foods, whether dairy, eggs, meat, poultry, or fish proteins—just like us, they absorb the energy from plants and it moves up the food chain. This also means that oils and fats extracted from well-cultivated foods—whether olive or flax, butter or cream,—can be replete with energetic potential too.

With the kitchen as my classroom, I discovered that, contrary to what some might assume, the etheric energy of food does not diminish when cooked—heat can be our ally, making the food easier to digest. In clinical practice it can be seen how even when a patient is in a weakened state, food imbued with energy can support the healing potential; it is the quality of food that matters, that can turn around the weakened condition, and in fact the simple foods are the best.

In the new world order of high-yield farming and chemical processing, the natural healing potential of food has turned to the opposite: low-vitality foods that lead us to overeat as our bodies try to satisfy their need for minerals and energy. As described in chapter 2, if food has incoherent energy patterns due to interferences, it can disturb the endocrine system, create fatigue and low vitality, and create the conditions for disease. (The disturbance extends beyond us: Intensive agriculture is also extremely damaging to ecosystems, causing chemical runoffs in water that disturb the balance of life in waterways and oceans and emitting noxious gases that can contribute to climate change.)

It is no coincidence that Dr. Parcells's pioneering analysis began in the 1950s, the beginning of her era of "better living through kitchen chemistry." Prior to the postwar period, most food was cultivated in chemical-free ways and was naturally imbued with etheric energy. Once the industrial food era began, Dr. Parcells began to counteract its influence in her own way through not only eating a chemical-free diet rich in healing potential but also mastering what she called "kitchen chemistry": If we could not avoid the contaminants, or if organic foods were not available, Dr. Parcells taught how to cleanse food using the Clorox Food Bath to clear contaminants from nonorganic produce, neutralizing the chemicals and allowing the food's own energy to flow.

Eighty years after Dr. Parcells's research on food's subtle energetics began, we are in a moment of reckoning. I believe that it takes thirty years of the restoration of soil through nonchemical farming to restore soil to its vital state. And while the awakening around food's impact on health is accelerating, our reality is that the majority of food on offer is not at its optimal energy level.

## Our Modern Conundrum

One of the first questions I ask every patient is "What are you eating for breakfast, lunch, and dinner?" In asking for a rundown of the average day, I am not trying to ascertain whether they are strictly sticking to a certain food doctrine or ideology. Nutrition is an individual matter and we can fine-tune almost any choice of diet and optimize it for each person's body, be they vegetarian, meat eater, pescatarian, paleo, ketogenic, or Ayurvedic in philosophy—or something else entirely.

Rather, I am looking for the obvious things, such as whether they are eating processed foods, excessive sugar and heated oils, and hard-to-digest baked goods. I am also looking for the less obvious: Is their diet a vital one? Is their food organically raised with healing potential? And what is their body doing with the food they are eating?

The answers that come are diverse—a mirror of our collective eating habits. Some people are eating out three meals a day or grabbing food on the run; others are subsisting on supersmoothies or meal-replacement bars, plus supplements to replace food. Others may be committed to paleo or vegan or raw-food paths, at times going to extremes of excluding certain food groups, while some zip around from one new food trend to another. Some feel confident about their diet, many do not, and even while a good number are making conscious choices to ensure good nutrition—putting thought and care into most meals—they may still find it challenging to consistently cook food at home for themselves.

The commonality across the board? Unless they have already taken steps to buy organic food, most of their meals, drinks, and snacks have low vitality. Meanwhile, it is fairly standard to discover a glaring lack in their diet of enough fresh and cooked vegetables, fruits, and herbs—the foods that would most support their vital force.

As a practitioner of subtle medicine, my goal is to gently remind each person that nature has its own pattern that works in harmony with us. We do not have to try so hard to "raise" or "better" that pattern through radical programs or cocktails of excess superfoods.

But neither can we cheat or hack the pattern too much—say, by guzzling every good ingredient for the day in one blended drink or consuming our biggest meals late at night, when we finally sit down and stop moving. What is more helpful is to return to *simplicity* by honoring basic laws that have been a basis of healing for millennia and that exist to help us flourish through our food.

Natural laws are universal principles that govern how nature works and life grows. A natural law could be as simple as the fact that plants need a certain amount of water and sunlight, and that the stronger the sun, the more water is required. When it comes to caring for our bodies, there are similar basic principles guiding our body's function. Over the years, my own understanding of natural laws of eating has come to include the consideration of food's etheric energetic potential. When followed, and used in tandem with the other principles of self-care, these principles can not only help us find our ideal weight but also help us to cut through the confusing nutritional landscape and stay connected to the subtle nourishing power of food.

Damian was a busy entrepreneur who thrived in his fast-paced, demanding job. But when he came to Light Harmonics, energetically his nervous system was near exhaustion. His skin looked dull and the quality of his etheric field was gray. He shared that he had adapted to a norm of poor sleep, elimination issues, fatigue during the day, and quite frequent moments of nausea but for some time had chalked it up as the inevitable side effects of reaching his late thirties and working hard.

Damian's lifestyle involved eating out two to three times a day, grabbing coffee and lunch from delis and takeout spots, dining out with clients or friends, and using post-workout power bars and energy drinks for fuel, or elaborate smoothies made with everything but the kitchen sink thrown in. His symptoms were expressing how too much poor-quality, overheated restaurant food had left his digestive force struggling to extract nutrients and energy from food and had diminished his ability to detoxify. The fat-rich, complicated smoothies weren't helping things; he was just putting expensive ingredients into a broken system.

Damian committed to six weeks of simplification by following the Liver-Cleansing Diet, with baths and homeopathy as support to relieve interferences and stress. Skeptical at first of his new morning breakfast—the Liver-Cleansing Drink uses garlic, ginger, and olive oil to nourish and stimulate the organs of detoxification and elimination—he soon became a convert. "It's like the world looks different," he told me. "I feel fresher; my life looks fresher!" The fog of congestion was starting to evaporate and his vitality was beginning to come back. His need for caffeine diminished too. The more he took control of his food, the more his symptoms began to subside; he looked "fresher" and brighter too. An added bonus: Damian fell in love with his kitchen, initiating what is now a long-standing practice of cooking and entertaining at home on a weekly basis. Damian's restaurant days were not done—eating out was still part of his lifestyle—but he chose eateries that fit into his food program.

## Conscious Nutrition Guidelines

### 1. When Possible, Eat Foods Sourced Locally

We used to categorize animals as carnivore, omnivore, and so on. A new buzzword fits my credo the best: *locavore*. Whenever possible, buy fresh, organic, and local. From an energetic perspective, growing and picking our own food is the ideal—of course, food grown in soil that we lovingly tend, water, and weed ourselves has the fullest potential of all! But unless a garden or a community plot is available, as well as significant free time, this may not be within reach. So do the best you can and source your food from farmers' markets and organic food markets whenever possible. No matter where you shop, look for the freshest seasonal produce you can find. If possible, cook homemade foods as a habit, using organic produce—or fresh conventional vegetables cleansed according to the instructions of the Clorox Food Bath—as well as whole, unadulterated grains, proteins, and quality fats as much as possible. If you can, grow something yourself, such as tomatoes and lettuces in a planter, herbs in a window box, or sprouts on the kitchen counter. Try to avoid using boxed or packaged foods, even if made from "whole foods," and when you do buy packaged foods, look for glass packaging instead of aluminum or plastic.

While good sources make all the difference, it's important not to get anxious or fanatical about the pursuit of them, for stress defeats the purpose. By following the protocols in Part Two, by enjoying diversity in your diet, rotating your foods according to season, and using methods for clearing interference and contamination when necessary, you can easily enjoy a diet that is safe and good for you.

There are more benefits to eating this way: When we support organic and local food, we are making a better choice not only for ourselves but also for our environment.

## 2. Face "Vegetable-Forward"

In busy lives filled with work, travel, caring for others, and meeting responsibilities, it becomes all too easy to forget to include fresh vegetables at meals, despite the best of intentions. Protein foods and carbohydrates are quicker and easier to source—restaurants make proteins and starches the main dishes on the menu, and how often are fresh and cooked vegetables the grab-and-go option at an airport or office snack bar?

But it's important to shift vegetables from supporting act to central player. While all the food groups are essential, including proteins, fats, and carbohydrates, from a point of view that integrates the physical and the subtle, *vegetables* are the foods that truly unlock harmonic health.

We need vegetables or fruits with our meal for multiple reasons: The mineral salts that they contain help us to digest proteins, which is why we include vegetables with a protein. The mineral salts in the water of the vegetable or fruit acts as a digestive juice, supporting the breaking down of food while hydrating our bodies too—they are the unsung heroes supporting our physical-etheric body in many ways. Of course, the bounty of protective antioxidants, vitamins, and other phytochemicals in fruits and vegetables also work harmoniously to support the function of the body and serve to combat damage that free radicals from toxins can unleash. The fiber in plant foods helps to sweep waste materials bound with bile out of the colon, including the excess cholesterol, used hormones, and chemicals and metals. The fiber also acts as a prebiotic that fuels the activity of the beneficial probiotics in the gut, which are so important in resisting parasites and countering inflammation. These probiotics—which are particularly enhanced by eating vegetables—also transform lignans, compounds in plants, into a plant hormone that protects women from the potential damage of excess estrogen. When vegetables are included in significant amounts, we find that the need for supplements and digestive enzymes diminishes—supported with what it needs, the body can be its own pharmacy and do the work for us.

My guideline is to give 80 percent of the space on the plate to plant foods, vegetables and herbs, or fruits. From a yogic point of view, vegetables, fruits, and herbs are replete with sattvic qualities. *Sattva* is one of the three *gunas* or universal forces of consciousness, and it is a quality of love, awareness, connection, and peace. Sattvic foods purify the body and calm the mind and help us to experience a harmonious state of health. We want to include a bounty of them each day.

## MEAT OR VEGETABLES? THE ANSWER IS BOTH

Some are surprised that given my reverence of plant foods, the Harmonic Healing philosophy does not stipulate following a vegetarian diet. Clinically, I have observed that a vegetarian diet works well for some—but not for all. I see this largely as relating to one's family constitution, geological location, occupation, and upbringing. If vegetarian eating has not been adhered to from a young age, or even been established in one's family lineage, the body can struggle to get the protein it requires, for plant protein requires more digestive force than meat. (The cow has assimilated the plant food by chewing the grass to make protein; the proteins in plant foods are more difficult to digest and not as easily available as those in meat, which is already a protein; our bodies must process the plant food in order to make it into a complete protein.) Meat can be a helpful protein source for healing and rebuilding when our digestion is weak. A diet well chosen for your needs can be your medicine, and the path of conscious nutrition includes grateful awareness of the origin of our foods. I like to say, don't focus solely on what you put into your mouth; pay attention to what comes out of your mouth—kindness and loving words—and you will create a field of health.

## 3. Eat with the Seasons

Seasonal foods are gifts from the earth. They don't merely excite us with the pleasure of the new; they are filled with goodness that supports us to stay well, during the season they grow. Even so, the fairly subtle nature of seasonal change gets easily overlooked in a globalized world, where foods are shipped across borders year-round, arriving at times that nature would normally not deliver them. Conscious nutrition involves noticing the seasonal changes in our local food sources—noting what's affordably in abundance in the produce section or, better yet, what's brimming on the farm stand—and then using them in our everyday eating to attend to the shifting needs of our bodies. The oft-quoted maxim "As above, so below; as within, so without" means that our internal environment adjusts in sync with shifts in weather and seasons, and our body clock follows rhythms of day and night; just like nature, we fluctuate. Our body's "fire" tends to get higher in the hotter weather and longer days of summer, making cooling foods such as cucumbers and zucchini more helpful; and as the heat diminishes, cold weather and longer nights take over, making warming and grounding foods appropriate, such as sweet potato, rutabaga, beets, carrots, and squashes, as well as beans. Spring vegetables like radishes, asparagus, and artichokes have both bitter and astringent (drying) tastes, which are wonderful for cleansing, along with bitter dandelion greens and chicory, which cleanses the liver and wakes up the digestion at a moment when all nature is bursting into renewal. And when spring becomes summer again, the cleansed digestive force can begin to rebuild in preparation for the colder weather again. Summer vegetables and fruits like tomatoes, peaches, and apricots support the rebuilding of our digestive process in warmer times through their watery nature. From an energy perspective, these foods have a clear resonance with our bodies' needs as they shift and change at different times of year. You might notice how uplifted you feel when foods are served according to the season.

The elements in our body can also change as if mirroring the world around us—for example, the winds of fall can aggravate the air quality within, and wet, damp weather can push our water and earth elements to an extreme—in Ayurvedic terms, we say they become aggravated or deranged, and this is often the beginning of imbalance that leads to symptoms within. Our diet is the simplest way to bring support in these times; when we choose foods with properties that soothe aggravation and restore balance, such as raw salads and cooling fruits in summer and heartier cooked plant foods like root vegetables, beans, and grains in fall and winter, we can help ourselves stay in sync and experience harmonious function within.

Take this awareness one level deeper, and we can begin to tune in to how our individual tendencies actually differ from one person to the next, just as climate differs from one area to the next. Most traditional medicines classify individuals according to body types that have certain elements more "in the fore" or predominating than others. One person is governed by fire, the next by air, and the next by water, in combinations that typically have two elements competing for the top spot. Getting to know our personal type is the *second* level of subtle medicine and is best performed with the help of a trained practitioner who can help take care of areas of weakness before they cause disturbance. But we can start tuning in to this by noticing when we tend to feel extremes in our system, like ebbs and flows of heat or ungrounded, airy sensations in the body or mind. Our intuition and our senses can often guide us right—making cucumbers appealing when we feel overheated or denser, oilier foods soothing when we're ungrounded. Nature teaches that we are individuals who live with fluctuation and change, and for this reason diet, like life, is not one-size-fits-all.

## 4. Combine Foods in Simple Ways

Avoiding improper combinations that place undue burden on digestion is a key to longevity and health. Poor digestion can be the beginning of a health challenge. One of the causes can be the way we combine foods in a meal. While proteins require the digestive juices of mineral-filled vegetables to digest, starchy carbohydrates like grains require pancreatic enzymes, which can act to neutralize the digestive process needed for protein. Eating proteins and hard starches such as wheat at the same time, therefore, adds unnecessary challenge to the digestion. Fruits, meanwhile, digest well with proteins or grains, which is why a bowl of oatmeal and berries can be a delicious and nurturing breakfast, although some very quick-to-digest fruits like melon are best eaten alone.

At a more nuanced level, awareness of food combining becomes an awareness of how to *balance* a meal. Subtle medicines also teach that the different "tastes" provided by nature—sweet, salty, sour, pungent, bitter, and astringent—exist to balance the elements within our bodies. In general, we want to include all tastes in our diet, which we can encourage through vegetables, fruits, herbs, and spices and by avoiding getting into a rut of overly repetitive and exclusive diets. Tastes can also be used therapeutically to support organs in need, and in Part Two you will discover how the morning Liver-Cleansing Drink and bitter greens with your meals will do that. You benefit from basic food-combining knowledge even if you pay heed to only one foundational concept: Eat simply with uncomplicated food combinations for easier digestion.

## 5. Use Proper Methods of Preparation

When you cook with an awareness of energy, you find yourself preparing foods that honor the energy they contain and also honor the strength of your body's digestive fire. Slower, low-heat methods help to ensure the healing constituents of foods are best retained; they also preserve the flavors. Cooking can actually make food's vital energy *more* available, not less, by helping to break down the food for better digestion. When it comes to food's subtle energy, either the vitality is there from the growing stages or it is not—and as long as cooking methods are not damaging (like high heat and frying), the etheric energy field will persist during the cooking process.

Furthermore, not every body has a strong enough fire to digest raw foods; the stomach is like a pot cooking on the stove. The fire in the stomach may not have the ability to digest raw foods; in this case, foods need to be cooked. It also becomes more difficult to digest an excess of raw foods in the winter—cooking food helps to stoke the digestive fire, and spices and herbs can be added to help the digestion further. When we cook with the low and slow method outlined in Part Two, and when the ingredients are combined in the proper ways, the energy of the food is more available. It is no wonder that long- and slow-simmering soups are a staple in every culture, used to stimulate digestion and to nourish us with the minerals that the liquid draws out from the vegetables or bones.

Preparation also involves a consideration of the senses. Traditional ways of cooking always emphasized caring for the way foods look and smell, because digestion begins with the eyes (the sensory organ associated with the liver) and the nose, which captures aromas and arouses the digestive response. Combining appealing colors in a dish, cutting the vegetables with care, enhancing with fresh herbs or colorful spices speaks to the yogic truth: Food appreciated and experienced through our senses is food that digests more easily. There's another simple reason to get in the habit of cooking our vegetables—cooking reduces the volume so we can digest larger amounts. And in situations when sanitation is not guaranteed, cooking makes food safer to eat. I usually recommend eating cooked foods in third-world and developing countries.

Other preparations of foods, such as sprouting seeds to cultivate tendrils of fresh sprouts, can bring us the nourishment of the growing forces, and naturally fermenting vegetables or dairy can provide the probiotics needed for good bacteria.

## 6. Honor the Act of Eating

The attitude and habits that surround eating are as important as the food itself. Eating has for many people become a haphazard act, occurring at inconsistent times or in a rushed or forced manner. For some the act is surrounded by struggle, conflict, or even shame. And the result is that too often we feel a separation from this source of nourishment—we are at odds with it. This is a loss, not just of pleasure we could have from eating, but because under stress, we lose the ability to absorb the nutrition and energy we could. Our culture makes food available 24/7, tempting us with shelves full of convenient, food-like substances, and sends challenging messages about the ways our habits and bodies "should" look, all of which can add to the disconnect from the benefits of simple food. But we can bridge that separation by treating our food and our bodies with respect, via small gestures that reconnect us to the sacredness of food.

We honor our food and our bodies when we eat in accordance with our body's needs and in sync with its rhythms, which in turn are governed by the rhythms of the earth. Eating meals at regular times, with minimal snacking in between and eating our biggest serving of protein early in the day when the digestive fire is highest help us to do this. So does refraining from eating between meals, unless we experience hypoglycemia, which makes it necessary to have frequent, small meals to keep blood sugar up. It is better to pause from eating after one meal is done; allow the body to do its work of digesting, let the efforts complete, and then we can add more food to the stomach, the pot cooking on the stove. And then at night when we sleep, we rest the digestion so the liver can repair. In this way we honor our body's extraordinary efforts.

## THE LIVER'S CLOCK

The liver has a twenty-four-hour rhythm that follows the twenty-four-hour rhythm of the earth. From 3:00 P.M. until 3:00 A.M. the liver accumulates glycogen as a result of carbohydrate metabolism. After 3:00 A.M. until 3:00 P.M., it releases stored glycogen into the blood for use as energy. The bile-secretion rhythm is the reverse. Its maximum activity is at 3:00 P.M. and minimum at 3:00 A.M. In this process, the liver and gallbladder work in a synchronized mechanical and spiritual way according to the laws of nature. This rhythm connects the physical and spiritual worlds. Since the maximum release of bile needed for fat digestion occurs at 3:00 P.M. if the main meal is taken after 6:00 P.M., fat digestion is hindered. It is better to have the higher-fat meals early in the day.

Most important, we can reframe our approach to our meals. With small gestures, we can turn any meal from a pit stop into a moment of gratefully receiving nourishment. Sitting down to eat and making space for the meal by putting concerns aside allows us to be more present with our food, and in that relaxed state, we absorb more of its goodness. Relaxing and not worrying so much about our diets, enjoying food rather than fighting it, is one of the most critical yet unacknowledged aspects of nutritional health. In my decades of practice, I have never ceased to be humbled by the ability of food that is cooked at home to heal.

Consider that the word *sacred* is related to the word *sacrament,* which is the term for holy food used in ceremony to connect us to our higher nature and to the greater field of consciousness of which we are a part. Eating with presence and reverence helps us feel more connected within. It also helps us feel more connected without: to other people, as we share food or give thanks for those who grew or made it; to our environment, the source of our food; to the elements that helped it to grow—the air, fire, water, and earth and the subtlest element, the ether, from which all other elements arise. Eating can be an act that unifies, and when we consume clean, whole food with appreciation, we can connect heaven and earth.

The legendary founder of macrobiotic eating, Michio Kushi, once said, "Peace begins in the kitchens and pantries, gardens and backyards, where our food is grown and prepared. The energies of nature and the infinite universe are absorbed through the foods we eat and are transmuted into our thoughts and actions." As a practitioner, I have come to see it is the universal energy carried in the food, and the quality of peace surrounding the experience of eating, that makes simple good food from clean sources *enough* to nourish and to heal. If we're lucky, we have experienced how a grandmother's soup made from garden ingredients can feel so good to the body and the spirit—and what Grandmother knew is that we don't have to "do" so much to our food when it has energy; it already tastes so good!

Peace is the secret behind multidimensional healing. Peace in our minds brings peace to our bodies and harmony to our whole selves. While it can be hard to stay in a peaceful mind-set throughout an average day, we can cultivate it three times, at least, through the attitude we bring to the kitchen or to the table, by putting our attention toward love, contentment, and thankfulness for what we have. Sometimes what is perfect is that we are communing with others around food. While good food is healing, *gratitude* for the good food is even more healing.

One of my patients and friend, the artist Marina Abramovic, is known for her provocative performance pieces. She relies on the conscious nutrition guidelines to intentionally and thoughtfully use vital foods, including nourishing cooked vegetables at each meal accented with spices and herbs, as her primary method of sustaining herself during her demanding projects. She calls the path of Harmonic Healing one of "simple, old-fashioned, putting yourself together" in a world that is constantly pulling us, to the point we can sometimes feel we are coming apart. The daily practice of giving energized food to a body that has good digestion and is clear of interferences supports her to stay present and embody her purpose of giving art to others. It's common sense. When we put high-grade fuel into a well-cared-for vehicle, it performs well, it breaks down less, we enjoy the journey of our life, and we radiate more of who we are, clear in our intention.

> Malia, a longtime yogi, came to her appointment struggling with a broken ankle that was not healing easily. She was in pain, and angry that the injury was not healing after many months. She was a vegetarian who ate many of her meals in a community setting, and these meals had become rather homogenous, with more than a few processed vegetarian foods as well as quick-to-make starches and large, hard-to-digest beans that her liver was not processing well. In the community kitchen, the cookware and serving dishes were all made of aluminum. At home, busy Malia froze meals for everyday use and forgot to eat fresh foods full of vitality at their peak ripeness.
>
> The energy of Malia's etheric field was weak, and this was impeding her healing. She was in a protein deficit due to the lack of good-quality protein and minerals from ample fresh vegetables, and furthermore, parasites were interfering with absorption of food. Her body did not have enough re-

serves to draw from. To help get Malia out of this rut, I told her small amounts of well-chosen meats would help her re-build. After careful consideration, she decided to gratefully add meat, broth, and fish to her repertoire for a few months while also becoming more involved with sourcing fruits and vegetables locally. Malia began on the Liver-Cleansing Program, which cleared the way for her body to better di-gest her food, and with her new diet, she began to see her innate strength return, and her ankle healed nicely.

Malia came to see the ankle injury as an invitation to renew her relationship with food, seeing conscious eating as a preventive measure that is nutritional and spiritual and that has powerful reverberations, as she ensures the best health for herself, her children, and their children too.

## Putting It All Together: Connecting the Invisible Dimensions of Health

My hope is that the knowledge shared in Part One has illuminated some of the possibilities influencing how you are feeling and familiarized you with some of the possibilities for resolving symptoms you may have. I use the term *possibilities* deliberately, for the truth is that health is not always an exact science in which action A always leads to result B. We are all individuals with our different constitutions, physical, emotional, and mental tendencies, and past experiences. Healing is a combination of science and art, in which a practitioner acknowledges the whole pic-ture of the patient's physical and subtle realms and looks for connections throughout all of it.

Health is a dynamic state; it is a *process,* and there is a humility to it: We engage in the process through our will, knowing that if we want health, we need to take care of ourselves on a day-to-day basis. Some-times challenges come up that are uncomfortable and difficult, but they very often end up teaching us something about ourselves—our tenden-cies and weaknesses, our ways of handling things, and even who we are and why we are here. The process of health inevitably looks a little different for each person, because each one of us is like a snowflake with a unique pattern.

Nevertheless, in today's world we all start at the same place by attending to the maintenance of our body—our vehicle for the journey of life. We maintain it the best we can to ensure well-functioning systems—digestive, immune, circulatory, respiratory, reproductive, elimination, and nervous systems—a clear mind, and fluidly moving emotions and the fortitude in our muscular and skeletal system that allows the vehicle to take us where we are meant to be. This basic maintenance cannot be side-stepped, even if our particular proclivity might be to immerse ourselves in what we consider to be "higher-level" practices like yoga, meditation, and prayer. All those things can create magic, but to *sustain* the magic in the everyday, we want to clean the filters, change the oil, check the spark plugs, tune up the engine, and improve the grade of the fuel! We do this primarily by taking care of the hardworking liver, which in turn helps the engine of our entire digestive system to function better, helps the "drains" of the lymph to stay clear, and gives relief to the endocrine glands. We also look to alleviate some of the pollution and shock in the etheric body, which can disrupt the energy flow. The methods for doing this and the lifestyle for maintaining this are what you will learn in Part Two.

It can be remarkable how much better we feel when our vital force is stimulated and nourished with etheric energy. The spark of life is lit again; the body's reserve energy is strong, allowing its healing potential to move freely. Reinvigorating our natural potential in this way helps us to rediscover a faith in our own ability to be well and a trust in our bodies' innate ability to heal. Touching this place of understanding is the beginning of attaining wholeness and peace, and of living with greater consciousness of ourselves and our connection to the whole. This was my earliest lesson from yoga, and it continues to inform everything that I do as an energy medicine practitioner today. When our bodies are harmoniously in balance, we radiate brightly.

Let's now discover how to help you reignite the spark!

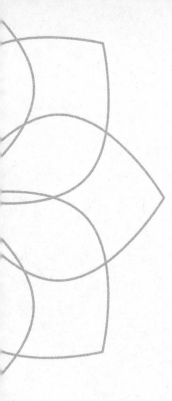

**PART TWO**

# Restoring Your Vitality and Health

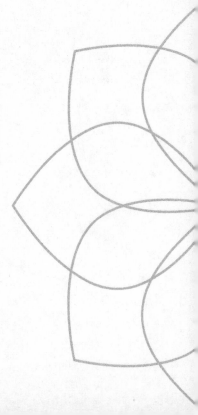

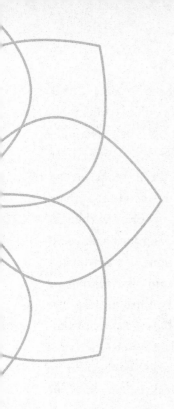

Chapter 6

# The Harmonic Healing Liver-Cleansing Program

Now that the principles of balanced living in our modern world are understood, it is time to look at daily practices that we can use to neutralize modern-day interferences. Everything you've learned up to this point is the backbone of the Liver-Cleansing Program that follows, which has been time tested in my practice to restore the body's natural levels of vitality.

The program involves two aspects: the Liver-Cleansing Diet, a food-based program that creates stress-free liver cleansing, and therapeutic baths to neutralize interferences at the cellular level. While the idea of detoxifying baths may be new to you, you are encouraged to include them, as they ease congestion in the etheric body. If you do not have a bathtub, or if there is a health restriction preventing you from taking a bath, the Liver-Cleansing Diet on its own is capable of supporting your new path to vitality.

# How the Harmonic Healing Program Works

One of the liver's primary functions is to metabolize: proteins, carbo-hydrates, and fats. Yet it needs support to do this; what I find today is that most people are not metabolizing food through their liver. The six-week program is intended to help correct congestion in the liver. The program is divided into two parts. The first three weeks involve following the Strict Liver-Cleansing Diet, which eliminates foods that I have found to slow down liver function. The diet is supported with liver- and gallbladder-cleansing foods that are prepared using low-heat cook-ing methods; the meals comprise simple combinations of high-quality protein, vegetables, fruit, and cold-pressed extra-virgin olive oil that are quite easy to put together. On this diet, you will be introduced to the Liver-Cleansing Drink as a choice for breakfast. This drink is recom-mended for at least the first three weeks of the cleansing program, and you may continue it throughout the six weeks, as many patients do (in fact, many continue to use it as a daily cleansing breakfast long after the cleanse ends).

After three weeks on the strict diet, you will shift to the second phase of the program, the Modified Liver-Cleansing Diet, which includes whole grains, legumes, and potatoes. The modified phase offers an abun-dance of delicious things to eat—including a variety of breakfast choices. It is so satisfying that many patients use it as a baseline for their ongoing lifestyle, veering off it only for special occasions. One caveat: If you are vegetarian or vegan, you are recommended to follow the modified diet's lunch and dinner protocols for all six weeks to ensure you have enough food options, while using the Liver-Cleansing Drink for the first three weeks, and longer if desired.

The program is designed to cleanse your liver and to give the sup-port and rest that the liver needs to cleanse the toxic burden from poor diets and overindulgences. It also guides you in preparing, cooking, and eating foods that heal and in forging the path for continuing with this as a way of life. After six weeks of eating simple foods, the taste buds begin to crave the foods that best support health. The body knows what it wants!

## CUSTOMIZING THE DIET

If you are seeking to lose weight, continue on the Strict Liver-Cleansing Diet for six weeks. Conversely, if you are concerned about losing weight or are a vegetarian who will need protein from legumes to thrive on this plan, you may choose to be on the Modified Liver-Cleansing Diet for six weeks.

Though it is appealing to imagine that six weeks of a cleansing diet each year can counterbalance forty-four weeks of unsupportive eating and living, my clinical experience shows that this does not typically work. True health is a process, not an outcome, and is best achieved slowly over time by clearing the layers of congestion and interference as they arise. For example, if the intestines have been aggravated and inflamed for some time by a bacteria or even candida, we can expect this to take more than several months to resolve. The approach is to take it one step at a time, moving gradually in order to stimulate the body's self-healing mechanisms and to support the vital force. When we maintain a day-to-day lifestyle of good diet and therapeutic baths, we maintain the conditions for the body to engage in a deeper state of physical, emotional, and mental balance.

Importantly, all the ingredients used in the program are natural foods or kitchen staples that may be found at your local stores. The program does not require the purchase of specialty items or expensive supplements. Fundamental to Harmonic Healing is understanding the restorative power of nature—radiant vitality, renewed energy, and ongoing resiliency to the challenges of our daily life. Do not be fooled by the simplicity of these protocols, however. By tending to the foundational requirements of detoxification and digestion through simple protocols, you are laying the groundwork for restoring your body's ability to heal.

At the mental and emotional level, cleansing the liver for six weeks with this program can have many effects. Thinking processes can become more clear, and negative emotions and aggravated temper, anxiety, and depression can begin to dissipate. When the liver is less inflamed, our mental and emotional state is less constricted with adversity and anger. Though there are never any guarantees, when liver function and digestion improve, reproductive-health issues like disruptive PMS, irregular periods, hot flashes in menopause, issues with the ovaries and uterus, and in some cases difficulty conceiving can begin the process of resolving themselves. Very often, clearing the liver revives the vital force, and that starts the process of regaining our balance as we begin to metabolize our food.

## ASSESSING YOUR READINESS TO BEGIN

### IS THE LIVER-CLEANSING PROGRAM RIGHT FOR YOU?

Children and pregnant or breast-feeding women should not do the complete program; however, they can follow the Modified Liver-Cleansing Diet and enjoy using all the recipes and ingredients it includes. Both groups should be careful to consume slightly more protein than the moderate portions advised here because of the body's greater needs for growth and development. Children and pregnant or breast-feeding women should not use the Liver-Cleansing Drink, but instead drink freshly squeezed orange or grapefruit juice at breakfast and then follow with one of the breakfasts from the modified diet, such as oatmeal and berries or a vegetable egg omelet. If you are over three months pregnant, refrain from the baths entirely (in the first trimester, tolerably hot baths are okay); nursing mothers should wait until after breast-feeding is finished to do any detoxifying practices such as the baths, so that toxins are not discharged via the breast milk. Children can do detoxifying baths with half the dosages of the ingredients listed.

If you are currently undergoing chemotherapy, you may enjoy the foods here, but please wait to engage in the full cleansing program until after your treatment is complete, as the baths can neutralize chemicals and therefore interfere with the medications used in the chemotherapy treatment.

The following questions will help you to identify whether your liver and gallbladder are experiencing overwork, as they point to some of the most common symptoms that can result.

Is your energy lower than you'd like it to be, or do you find it challenging to meet the demands of daily life?

Do you regularly experience digestive issues, nausea, bloating, gas, or abdominal discomfort?

Are your stools especially light brown, yellow colored, or unformed (which indicates suppressed bile)?

Do you get headaches or migraines?

Do you have skin issues such as rashes, acne, or pimples?

Do you have poor appetite—or get hungry soon after meals, with an insatiable desire to eat?

Do you have sugar cravings?

Do you have low hormone levels or reproductive issues?

Is your sleep disrupted, or do you have trouble falling asleep?

Do you think more slowly or have brain fog at times?

Do you have anxiety or feel depressed?

Do you have lack of enthusiasm or low esteem?

**Candida Spotlight:** If you have any of the symptoms described in Chapter 3 that are indicative of candida overgrowth, it is suggested that you do the Candida Protocol, page 150, alongside the Strict Liver-Cleansing Diet. The Candida Protocol is very similar to the Liver-Cleansing Diet, but also helps the body to clear candida by removing sweet fruits, fermented foods and drinks, and any sugars you might be tempted to eat that feed the yeast. If after reading about the symptoms you are not sure if candida is a pressing concern, you can follow the six-week Liver-Cleansing Program and assess how you are feeling afterward. You can also talk to your doctor about getting a test for candidiasis.

## The Liver-Cleansing Diet

The Liver-Cleansing Diet helps to cleanse and revitalize the liver by removing foods that have congesting or aggravating effects and filling the diet with foods that support the functions of the liver. In so doing, it counters what I have observed to be the primary causes of malnutrition, which include wrong food combinations, foods that are low in minerals and high in chemicals and hormones, and processed, overrefined foods laden with preservatives, food colorings, and additives. These foods interfere with the natural balance of our etheric field and impede the digestive organs' ability to assimilate nutrients and energy. A primary goal in these six weeks is to purchase fresh, good-quality food that whenever possible is organic or biodynamic. Locally raised, farm-stand foods grown without chemicals, even if not officially certified organic, are good choices too (some nonchemical growers do not have certification). If you are unsure of a food's provenance, you can cleanse any lingering chemicals with the Clorox Food Bath (page 144).

Anytime you change your diet, a little understanding of the principles goes a long way in motivating you to stick with it. On this program, certain foods will be eliminated for six weeks and others prioritized, in order to gently restore the liver's ability to metabolize proteins, carbohydrates, and fats. Here's why:

- When the liver is not processing fats, symptoms such as nausea, headaches, insomnia, abdominal distention or bloat, and acid reflux can exist. When we eliminate cooked oils and nuts and use unheated extra-virgin olive oil to help it "flush," the liver gets a rest and can start to process fats again.

- When the liver is congested, it almost always struggles to process carbohydrates, leading to weight gain and blood-sugar issues. On the program, we eliminate hard-to-process sugars and carbohydrates such as baked goods, whole grains, and white potatoes during the strict phase, in order to rest and repair the liver until it begins to process better. While whole grains and potatoes are added back during the Modified Liver-Cleansing Diet, baked goods and sugars remain off the diet for the entire six weeks.

- Good-quality proteins are used throughout the six weeks, balanced with vegetables and fruit. Vegetarians and vegans can do the Modified Liver-Cleansing Diet for the whole six weeks in order to include legumes and whole grains.

- Your only added fat source (beyond what naturally occurs in the foods) is cold-pressed, extra-virgin olive oil, which is used as a condiment after food is cooked or in dressings and dips for salads. High-quality flaxseed oil can be used similarly. The Liver-Cleansing Diet avoids heating oils while ensuring that we get enough fats to nourish the body and to promote a healthy nervous system. When oil is heated, the molecules change from round to jagged, which can be an irritant to the liver, can interfere with digestion, and can cause inflammation in the body. By using unheated, extra-virgin olive oil we get the benefit of its wonderful liver and nervous system support. You will learn techniques for cooking vegetables and proteins without heating oils on direct high heat in chapter 8.

## Foods to Eliminate

For all six weeks of the Liver-Cleansing Diet, eliminate the following:

**All fried foods, whether homemade, restaurant prepared, or packaged, including chips.** This can include obvious fried foods such as French fries and fried chicken, as well as tempura, stir-fries, and breaded and fried appetizers and entrées.

**All oils except raw, unheated, cold-pressed extra-virgin olive oil or high-quality flaxseed oil used after cooking or on salads.** One of the easiest ways to relieve liver stress is to focus on good fats and limit the heating of oils, which may have been aggravating and irritating your liver. We also avoid the rancid and inflammatory effects of industrial seed oils. Oils can be hard to avoid when dining out, but there is usually a best choice that you can make on a menu that focuses on simply prepared vegetables and lean protein that is grilled, roasted, or in a stew or ragout. After the cleanse, you will be able to start cooking with a wider array of natural fats, as your liver will be able to metabolize and digest them again.

**All sugar and corn syrup, and all processed foods with preservatives and additives.** This is the obvious omission. The body has a hard time knowing what to do with these ingredients. Sugars overburden our pancreas and feed the candida that can be present. Minimal amounts of raw honey, grade-A maple syrup, or molasses can be used in the program if candida is not present. Additives and processed foods are difficult for our liver to digest and should be eliminated. We were designed to digest food in as close to its natural state as possible and without man-made chemicals.

**All dairy products.** Dairy, in its pasteurized and hormone-filled form in the West, has become an inflammation-causing food and is difficult for the body to break down, especially when mixed with other foods. Excess dairy bogs down the digestion, and our inability to digest can create mucus and phlegm when dairy is combined with other proteins. When the liver and gallbladder are working well after the program is complete, heavy cream as a fat and raw dairy products as protein can be used if they cause no discomfort.

**All grains and white potatoes.** Grains (including corn and corn-based products and pasta), as well as white potatoes, are starches that break down to sugar. They are eliminated during the strict phase. (The body breaks down sweet potatoes more slowly due to their higher fiber content, unlike white potatoes, which can spike the blood sugar. This is why sweet potatoes and yams are allowed during the strict phase.) Quinoa, a fairly digestible seed that has the feel of a grain once cooked, can be enjoyed throughout the six weeks. In weeks 4–6, you may add back whole, well-cooked grains such as brown and wild rice, oats, millet, and corn tortillas, as well as buckwheat soba noodles, whole-grain pasta, and white potatoes. Those seeking to lose weight should continue avoiding all whole grains and white potatoes during weeks 4–6.

> The inclusion of grains and white potatoes is the primary differ-ence between the Strict Liver-Cleansing Diet, (weeks 1–3) and the Modified Liver-Cleansing Diet (weeks 4–6). Please note that if your blood sugar is low or you experience rapid weight loss, you may eat whole cooked grains, seeds, and potatoes dur-ing all six weeks.

**Bread, cookies, pastries, crackers, pretzels, and other baked goods.** A special mention for these products, which are typically made from grains—though not always, given the rise of gluten-free products, which use tapioca, nut flours, soy, and potato starch. Baked goods are high in starchy carbohydrates and many are filled with sugar, which we want to avoid while cleansing and thereafter reserve for special occasions. This is especially important when following a candida diet, for in addition to sugar, these products often contain yeast. Baked goods are eliminated for *all six weeks.*

**Nuts and seeds.** Why no nuts? It's not that nuts are bad; they are a great source of protein and fat, but only if our body can digest them. How-ever, nuts, including coconuts, are very concentrated sources of protein and fats—the phrase "hard as a nut" exists for a reason. They are difficult for the digestive juices to break down, especially in the high volumes in which they are ingested these days. Nuts and seeds and the products derived from them are eliminated in the Liver-Cleansing Program in order to help the liver and gallbladder to heal. This means that nut and seed butters, nut milks and creams, oils such as coconut oil and coco-nut manna, nut and seed flours, and nut and seed bars and snacks are completely eliminated for the first three weeks. Two exceptions to the rule are flaxseed and chia seeds, which are allowed throughout. (The teaspoon of ground flaxseed in the Liver-Cleansing Drink supports the liver, digestive system, and bowels.) Chia seeds are allowed because of their gelatinous nature and ability to hydrate us.

**Alcoholic beverages.** When cleansing the liver, we want to avoid drinking alcohol unless there is a special occasion. If you have candida, it is recommended that you choose a clear spirit like 100 percent agave tequila or distilled vodka instead of wine or beer, which are fermented. If you are not symptomatic with a candida overgrowth and there is a wedding, birthday, or other time for celebration, a glass of champagne or a fine old wine with your meal is certainly acceptable to celebrate with. It is not what you do once in a while but what you do on most days that makes a difference in regaining health.

**Pork; shellfish; crustaceans such as shrimp, lobster, and crabs; and bottom-feeding fish such as halibut, flounder, cod, and some species of shark.** Heavy metals sink to the bottom of the ocean and bottom-feeding fish will often be more contaminated by these metals. Pigs do not have sweat glands and have a tendency to be a more toxic meat. Avoiding these types of proteins during a cleanse is recommended.

## The Foods to Enjoy

For all six weeks of the Liver-Cleansing Diet, you may have all that you desire of the following foods:

**Meat and poultry, except for pork.** Strive to use meat or poultry that is organic and/or grass-fed, wild, or at the very least raised with no hormones added to feed or used in rearing. Consider using chicken, turkey, beef, bison, elk, and lamb. The simplest preparation is always best. Grilling, roasting, making soups, stews, or ragouts, or pan-searing or braising without oil contributes to successful liver cleansing. Sliced/packaged lunch meats or deli meats are not recommended because they are processed. Roasted turkey sliced off the bone or roast beef can be used during liver cleansing.

**Seafood (except for shellfish, shrimp, lobster, crabs, and bottom-feeding and farm-raised fish).** Seafood is a good choice for easy-to-digest protein. Enjoy it poached, baked, grilled, cooked in parchment paper, naturally cured (in the case of salmon), or as ceviche. I am always asked what kind of fish to use; wild Alaskan salmon seems to be the safest fish these days, and you can even trust it as sashimi, as long as it is fresh and wild. However, it is important to learn how to identify fresh fish. Fish should never smell fishy, and you should ask your fishmonger to let you smell it. It should be springy and a bit translucent, and the eyes must look clear. Ideally, avoid canned fish as much as possible during this time; if you need to use canned salmon, sardines, herring, or tuna, you can, but it is better to purchase in glass jars, such as Italian tuna paired with olive oil for a quick meal.

**Eggs.** Eggs are best enjoyed poached or soft-boiled, as these methods avoid heated oils and preserve the delicate nutrients best. A slow and low-heat scramble, fritatta, or omelet using a little ghee for the cooking fat is also delicious cooked with vegetables.

If you are unsure of the origin of your protein, use the Clorox Food Bath (page 144). This is especially important for fish from toxic waters and fish farms.

**Lentils and legumes.** Lentils of both European and Indian dal varieties and beans, including white beans, black beans, red beans, and kidney beans, are another protein source and especially good for vegetarians. Do not mix beans (such as in a three-bean salad), as each bean digests differently and it is best to keep things simple so as not to stress the digestive system. One type of bean or legume with plenty of vegetables works. Avoid processed soy products like tofu and tempeh. Homemade tofu was a staple in my vegetarian household, but the amount of time it takes to make really outweighs its benefits. If you can find a good Japanese restaurant that makes homemade, custardy tofu, then it is a treat to have occasionally. Try to use dry organic lentils and legumes, not canned. Note that with dals and lentil soups, such as the ones listed in Chapter 8, you can easily add vegetables into the pot to make a complete one-dish meal.

**All vegetables, cooked or raw, including sweet potatoes, squashes, and beets (exception: white potatoes for first three weeks).** Include plenty of seasonal vegetables whenever you can, and use abundant servings of cooked and raw leafy greens frequently. Vegetables can be grilled, roasted, steamed, slow-cooked in soups or stews, or combined in salads. Olive oil can be used to season, along with herbs, lemon, and sea salt, after cooking. Fermented vegetables like sauerkraut and kimchi, as well as fermented soybeans in the form of miso paste, can be used in the program unless you are following the Candida Protocol. If you are seeking to lose weight, limit your intake of starchy vegetables such as roots and winter squashes during both phases of the Liver-Cleansing Diet, (strict and modified). If you are not purchasing organic vegetables and fruits, please refer to the instructions for the Clorox Food Bath, page 144.

## VEGETABLES BY THE SEASON

**SPRING:** Look for artichokes, asparagus, bitter greens like dandelion and escarole, scallions, and radishes.

**SUMMER:** Look for zucchini, tomato, green leafy vegetables, celery, cucumber and peppers, baby bok choy, and baby beets and their leaves.

**FALL:** Look for root vegetables of all kinds, including yams, beets, parsnips, turnips, rutabaga, carrots, kohlrabi, celeriac, broccoli, kale, cabbage, and brussels sprouts.

**WINTER:** Look for winter squashes like pumpkin, acorn, spaghetti, buttercup, kabocha, and butternut.

**All fruits, raw, baked, or poached, (not dried) ideally in season and ripe.** When candida is an issue, and when seeking to lose weight, smaller portions are recommended, with a focus on fruits that are lower in sugars, such as citrus; summer tree fruits like cherries, apples, and pears; and berries, which tend to be eaten in smaller portions. If you are not concerned with weight, or seek to gain it, you can enjoy some tropical fruit like bananas, mangoes, and pineapple in moderation. Melons can be eaten alone as a meal (such as watermelon in summer for a light breakfast). Do not eat fruit that is not ripe because it is difficult to digest. Nature wants us to eat ripe fruit to get all its nutritional benefits from the sun.

## FRUIT COMBINING

Proper fruit combinations are important for digestion. Oranges, grapefruits, tangerines, and lemons are natural acid fruits and go nicely with other acid fruits such as pineapple and cranberries. Slightly acid fruits, such as apples, pears, plums, peaches, and apricots, can combine with acid fruits as well. Melons and berries should always be eaten alone.

| ACID FRUITS | SUB-ACID FRUITS | SWEET OR DRIED FRUITS |
|---|---|---|
| Oranges | Apples | Dates |
| Lemons | Pears | Figs |
| Grapefruits | Plums | Raisins |
| Limes | Peaches | Prunes |
| Cranberries | Grapes | Bananas |
| Pineapple | Apricots | |
| | Berries | |

Guidelines
- Acid fruits can combine with subacid fruits.
- Subacid fruits can combine with sweet fruits.
- Do not combine acid fruits with sweet fruits.
- Eat melons alone on an empty stomach.
- When fruits are not available ripe and in season, such as during the winter months, dried fruits can be incorporated.

All dried fruits need to be reconstituted or revived: Put them into cold water and bring it to a boil. Then turn off the flame, cover the pot, and let it sit overnight. Use the fruit the next day. The boiling kills all insects and parasites inside the fruit.

**Extra-Virgin Olive Oil.** We want to ensure we consume enough supportive fats on this program; therefore, we enjoy all the fats that naturally occur in the allowed meats, poultry, fish, and avocados; when we add fats to our food, we stick to fats the liver can easily process. Consume at least three tablespoons of olive oil or, as an alternative, flaxseed oil daily. (If you do not like the flavor of olive oil, flaxseed oil has a buttery flavor that merges nicely with lemon.) Your body will tell you if you need more or have had enough—it is normal to feel a craving for olive oil and fats at first, indicating you need more. Be sure to include some avocados for some fat too. I do not give exact amounts of olive or flaxseed oil to use; if you drizzle it according to taste, not drenching your food with oil, you will become comfortable with this style of eating and know how much your body needs. In addition, ghee (clarified butter) may be used to pop spices in recipes that call for this, and ghee and grapeseed oil can be used in place of heated olive or flaxseed oil if oil is required for low–heat sautéing. Both these fats can tolerate direct heat in a pan.

**Salt and seaweed.** The body needs salt to balance sugar in the blood; it controls the function of the adrenal glands and then controls the sugar balance in the body. I recommend using natural sea salt instead of common table salt because it is similar to the salt in our cells and lymphatic system. Seaweed also provides sodium but, more important, the use of seaweed daily is a protector against radiation. I often add a few large pieces of wakame to my soups—it is especially tasty in lentil soup.

## Clearing Food of Contaminants: The Clorox Food Bath

This technique was pioneered by Dr. Hazel Parcells to clear foods of contaminants and interferences in the home kitchen. You can use it anytime you are buying conventional (nonorganic) produce or are unsure of the origin of the food—for example, if you suspect it has been raised with chemicals. Please read the directions on page 159 to ensure you purchase the correct kind of Clorox.

### Instructions for Cleansing Food

Fill the sink with 1 gallon of cold water and add 1 teaspoon of regular Clorox.

Separate the foods into the following categories and soak them in the Clorox bath as follows:

Leafy vegetables, 5–10 minutes
Root and fibrous vegetables, 10–15 minutes
Thin-skinned fruits like berries, 5 minutes
Medium-skinned fruits like peaches and apricots, 10 minutes
Thick-skinned fruits like apples, 10–15 minutes
Citrus fruits and bananas, 15 minutes
Eggs, 20–30 minutes
Meat/poultry/fish, 10 minutes

After the soaking, transfer the foods to an equal amount of clean water and soak them for 5–10 minutes.

Let the food drain very well before placing them in refrigerator.

. . .

I have found that blessing food with intention also has the effect of raising the vibratory energy of food, and that a prayer or blessing spoken aloud and with pure intent has an even greater effect, because of the field of electromagnetic energy from our voice. Taking a moment before eating can be a ritual that is well worth incorporating into everyday life, reminding us to be present with our food and helping everyone at the table feel connected to one another.

## LIVER CLEANSING FOR VEGETARIANS AND VEGANS

If you do not eat fish, meat, eggs, or poultry, your meals will need more preparation time. A simple protein derived from animal food rebuilds the body more quickly than legumes can. It takes more energy to metabolize a grain or bean into a protein than a piece of meat, strange as this may sound. In the Liver-Cleansing Diet, vegetarians and vegans may use kitchari and dal as easy-to-digest protein dishes, as they contain small lentils or mung beans with the necessary spices to help digestion. In the case of kitchari, basmati rice is added to the lentils to form a complete protein, and this gentle and digestible meal is good to eat during the entire program of liver cleansing. Many staple vegetarian foods like larger beans (such as kidney, pinto, and white) are more difficult to digest, unless your digestion is working well or they are enhanced with a combination of spices or herbs. Note that for diversity, the vegetables can be changed according to season in these grain/legume stews. Following the Modified Liver-Cleansing Diet rules can be easily done by a vegetarian or a vegan.

## Drinks

- **WATER.** Drink two quarts of pure water daily, following the hydration guidelines on page 174.

- **COFFEE.** You may enjoy coffee daily, black, with no added milk, dairy substitute, or "bulletproof" fats at this time. If coffee is not your preference, a cup of black or green tea is acceptable.

### I CAN HAVE COFFEE?

Yes! The coffee bean is one of nature's bitter foods—one of the five tastes that the body requires to be in balance. Moderate use of coffee can help the system to cleanse; it is overindulgence in coffee that causes trouble. If you enjoy the mild stimulation of good-quality coffee, try to source organic coffee (or ask your roaster about the provenance of the beans, as farmers and roasters may not always have certification even when using no chemicals). High-mountain- and shade-grown coffee beans are preferable. Avoid coffee capsules, which can contain aluminum. A good stainless-steel espresso maker for espresso, a glass French press or a Toddy cold brew system are all easy to use; try to avoid coffeemakers made of plastic and aluminum. If you drink decaf, it is better to choose coffee that has been decaffeinated using the water extraction method.

## The Four Principles of Balanced Eating

Now that you know what to eat, let's talk about how to eat. These four principles will help you create simple meals, in your way and suiting your tastes.

## Principle 1: The 80:20 Ratio

This principle speaks to the balance between plant foods—vegetables, fruits, and herbs—and protein in each meal. The digestion of proteins is essential to the maintenance and repair of all cell tissue. Yet what many don't realize is that protein is concentrated and we don't need as much as people think. I advise that 20 percent of the plate or bowl be protein. The serving size should be about the size of the palm of your hand. The remaining 80 percent of the plate should be filled with vegetables or fruits. You may need more protein if you are doing hard physical labor, are an athlete, or are trying to build up the body (such as through weight lifting); but in general, abide by the 80:20 rule. If you are a meat eater and want to ingest more protein, then remember to also increase your vegetables to help process the larger quantities of protein. This principle of pairing protein with plenty of vegetables will ensure that the vegetable juices support the digestion of protein. When filling your plate or bowl with vegetables, aim to use a colorful, seasonal variety, and rotate your choices rather than relying on the same few vegetables all the time. "Finish" your dish by drizzling olive oil on your vegetables or salad.

## Principle 2: Proper Food Combining

For optimal digestion, follow these rules:

- **Do not combine different sources of protein in one meal.** Pick one type of meat, poultry, fish, legumes, or lentils. The one exception is egg, which mixes fine with other proteins or can be enjoyed on its own. When you return to dairy after liver cleansing, dairy or nuts should also be separate from other proteins—the very common combo of dairy and meat, such as in a cheeseburger, is difficult to digest.

- **Eat protein with vegetables, but separate it from gluten-containing grains like wheat, rye, and barley.** This includes all bread and pastries, cereals, and pastas. There's a learning curve as you adopt this rule, but soon

ou start to see how that (cheese-free) hamburger digests
ter without the bun. Similarly, oatmeal digests better
with cream (a fat) than with milk (a protein).

- **Eat grains, especially gluten-containing ones, with
  vegetables—for example, whole-grain pasta with a
  zucchini vegetable sauce.** I especially like farro pasta
  from Italy, brown rice pasta, quinoa pasta, and buckwheat
  soba noodles in the program. These items are always in my
  dry pantry.

- **In general, eat fruits and vegetables separately.** They
  serve different purposes. Fruits are for cleansing and are
  good for a start in the morning or quick energy at midday
  or as evening snacks. Vegetables are for building and
  supporting the digestive force. When making blended
  drinks, choose fruits or blended vegetables, but do not
  mix the two. The exceptions are apples, which digest
  with vegetables, and lettuce, which digests with fruits.

## Principle 3: Use Low and Slow Cooking Methods

Though we are told to cook at high heat and high speed in our busy
lives, I prefer low-heat, slow cooking. This not only helps to avoid overheating any fats but also protects the proteins. Proteins must be changed
into amino acids before they can be assimilated. There are twenty-two
amino acids that are essential to our health and eight amino acids that are
indispensable to life. Two of these amino acids regulate body functions
but are destroyed by high temperatures: tryptophan, which is a critical factor in our antibodies for our immune system, and lysine, which
stimulates the metabolic rate. Both of these indispensable amino acids
are destroyed in high-heat cooking. A slow-cooking methodology, using
lower temperature, is core to our approach.

## ADJUST CARBOHYDRATES TO YOUR BODY'S NEEDS

While all vegetables and plant-based foods are enjoyed in this diet, you will want to pick wisely between starchy vegetables and nonstarchy vegetables and low-sugar fruits and high-sugar fruits. One confusion lies in the understanding of carbohydrates—the food that the body turns into sugar for energy. While we recognize that bread, pasta, and potatoes are foods that are high in carbohydrates, we don't always recognize that all vegetables and fruits are carbohydrates, but in different percentages. Thus we want to choose wisely according to our body's needs and our desire to find balance. Choose low-carbohydrate vegetables and fruits for losing weight and high-carbohydrate ones for gaining weight. Carbohydrate counters are readily available online—keep one handy and be sure to keep the carbs from the starchy vegetables allowed on the program to under eighty grams daily if you seek to lose weight.

## Principle 4: Eat in Rhythm

It is preferable to get in the rhythm of eating at regular times and allowing two to three hours after meals for digestion to occur. Envision the stomach as a pot of rice cooking on the stove; to cook the food well, you first put in water, then add the rice, then if needed, add a little more water (for example, if you are thirsty while eating), and then . . . close the lid and allow the rice to cook! Just as a good chef doesn't add more ingredients or throw in cold water once the lid is on, so it is with our digestion. If after two to three hours you want a snack to get you through to the next meal, I suggest drinking water or a vegetable juice or eating a piece of fruit or guacamole with crudités.

Please honor the food by thoroughly chewing to mix the food with saliva and the enzymes it contains—this is the first phase of digestion that so often gets overlooked, especially if we are distracted or rushed at

Also take a moment before you start eating to appreciate the
you. I used to play a game with my children called "Who can
ce the longest?" We'd count fifteen, twenty chews or more.
ice is chewed well, the taste changes into a sweet flavor, and
ι loved the sweet taste as they chewed more.

---

## The Candida Protocol

Most people who have taken antibiotics have candida. Some
people's bodies live in balance with it, while others are overtaken by it and thus will want to attend to it. Clues that there is
a candida overgrowth may be feeling full or bloated after eating
carbohydrates; vaginal discharge; having a thick, white coating
on the tongue; and/or fungus lodged under toenails or finger-
nails (indicating that the fungus has become systemic). All these,
along with the symptoms described on page 59, indicate that you
should remain on the Candida Protocol until the symptoms have
cleared. The diet is essentially the Strict Liver-Cleansing Diet
with certain foods eliminated.

### ADDITIONAL ELIMINATED FOODS FOR CANDIDA PROTOCOL
- No fruit except low-carb fruits: grapefruit, berries,
  green apples.
- No fermented foods or drinks, including vinegar, miso,
  mustard, ketchup, soy sauce, barbecue or Worcestershire
  sauce, beer, wine, kombucha, kefir, or yogurt.
- No sugar.
- Special care should be taken to avoid moldy or aged
  foods.
- Dried fruits are concentrated sugar and should be
  eliminated.

- No processed or smoked meats, including ham, bacon, lunch meats, sausage, or hot dogs.
- Mushrooms are fungi and should be eliminated.

Include lots of fresh vegetables in your diet, and be sure to include garlic, onions, ginger, cabbage, broccoli, turnips, kale, and cauliflower, which support the detoxification of candida.

In addition, support daily detoxification with either olive-leaf extract or oregano oil, two herbal formulas that are easily found at any health-food store, used as directed on the bottles. When these formulas are coupled with the candida food program, my patients often report success. But note that the formulas on their own will not clear candida; they must be used in tandem with the diet.

The final important ingredient for candida clearing is patience. While the Liver-Cleansing Program is a six-week program, if you are clearing candida, you will likely be following the guidelines for longer. There is no easy way to say exactly how long the Candida Protocol must be followed, as this varies greatly from person to person, but several months is common and even up to a year is not unusual. Clearing fungus takes time, and since fungus is connected to the water element, it can create a lot of emotional cravings for carbohydrates and sugar, making dietary changes challenging. Although the Liver-Cleansing Diet and the Candida Protocol include plenty of wonderful and satisfying foods, the person burdened with candida often has strong cravings for sugar. Observe, breathe, and embrace all the good foods that you are allowed.

## The Strict Phase: Weeks 1–3

For the first three weeks you will follow the Strict Liver-Cleansing Diet. Breakfast is the Liver-Cleansing Drink, followed if you choose by Liver-Cleansing Tea. One cup of coffee is permitted, or black or green tea. Lunch and dinner are to be created from the "Foods to Enjoy" list, using the recipes and instructions included in this book, or simply assembled from the permitted foods. Be very mindful of the "Foods to Eliminate" list, and take care not to include any grains or white potatoes during these first three weeks.

Let's walk through one day on the program and see what this looks like.

## Breakfast

The Liver-Cleansing Drink is taken on an empty stomach as the first meal of the day. Its mix of grapefruit/orange, lemon, ginger, flaxseed, and cayenne, as well as—yes!—garlic and extra-virgin olive oil creates a unique drink that acts to "flush" the liver and gallbladder first thing in the morning after fasting all night long. The addition of garlic and olive oil to a morning drink is not nearly as strange-tasting as it sounds; the combination of sour, bitter, sweet, and pungent ingredients creates a flavorful, therapeutic drink. This is not an icy-cold "smoothie" but rather a blended cleansing drink. If you are embarking on the Liver-Cleansing Diet and know that you have excess acidity in your stomach—or if you experience burning in your stomach before or after eating or have been diagnosed with ulcers or reflux—please substitute the Green Liver-Cleansing Drink (page 212), which will also help the liver and gallbladder to clear, but without adding acidity from citrus, or choose the breakfasts listed for the Modified Liver-Cleansing Diet.

Think of this morning drink as breakfast; rather than chugging it down as you race out the door, please take your time with it, "chewing" each sip so that it begins to digest in the mouth. Since oxidation happens quickly once fruits or vegetables are liquefied, please drink your drink soon after blending, and start fresh the next day. The olive oil makes this drink very satisfying, so you will be able to wait at least two hours before eating any food afterward.

You may have your cup of black coffee or caffeinated tea after the drink, though for best results, follow the Liver-Cleansing Drink with the Liver-Cleansing Tea (page 212), which combines five spices and herbal ingredients that support the liver and the balance of the digestive fire—ginger, fenugreek, peppermint, fennel, and flaxseed—and a sixth optional ingredient, licorice root, into a delicious blend. This tea can also be used as a cleansing tea midmorning and midafternoon for additional support.

## Midmorning and Midafternoon Snack (Optional)

If you are hungry, you may have either one serving of fruit (a low-sugar fruit such as a green apple, a small bowl of berries, or a grapefruit if you are watching sugars), a vegetable juice, one of the blended vegetable drinks (page 216), a cup of warm Bone Broth (page 220), or crudités and guacamole. When drinking vegetable juices and drinks, take them on an empty stomach.

## Lunch and Dinner

When preparing lunch and dinner, go for easily digestible meals that are interesting to the senses, with lots of color, texture, and flavor. The overarching guideline is simplicity. You will select meat, fish, poultry, eggs, or legumes and pair with vegetables. You should prepare these foods simply, by steaming, grilling, braising, making a soup, or serving as a salad. Try to limit the number of different kinds of food eaten at one meal. If you are going to have several courses, such as when sharing a meal with others, put a little advance thought into it, ensuring you are still adhering to the food-combining rules throughout the meal.

These two main meals of the day can be created (or ordered) by following the simple formula: 1 protein + 2 or more vegetables + olive oil/ dressing (see page 258 for dressing recipes) as desired.

You can achieve this in various ways. In chapter 8, "Dr. Linda's Kitchen," you will find my family's favorite festive recipes that you can use throughout the cleanse. You can also combine the allowed ingredients in ways that you already know how to prepare or use the cooking instructions for basic proteins and vegetables to create very straightforward plates.

A sample week, including some of the meals I have suggested many times to patients and that I continue to use in my own kitchen today, is included as a template; this can serve as inspiration for you or as an actual eating plan, depending on the amount of structure you like. Many people do a mixture of both approaches—some days lunch is a piece of chicken or two soft-boiled eggs with mixed greens and half an avocado, while other days it's a warming bowl of lentil or dal soup with seasonal vegetables based on one of my recipes. There is no rule that the meal must be complicated or take a lot of time to prepare. Again, preparing and eating simple combinations of foods is the goal.

There may be days when it does not appeal to you to have a protein and two vegetables. Please note that you can have a sweet potato and steamed vegetables and skip the meat. Or perhaps all you want is a vegetable soup or a blended vegetable drink or a mug of broth on its own. Listen to your body. It is important that this diet fit into your life, and there is no rigid "right" way to do this. No matter how you assemble your plate, a drizzle of olive or flaxseed oil (or homemade olive oil–based salad dressing) may be added to your vegetables, and you can also choose to eat them plain, or as I like to call it, "naked"—as there is value in eating undressed, lightly steamed vegetables during cleansing! Try to consume beets two to three times a week, and make sure green vegetables, and especially bitter greens, are consumed daily. During this phase, you are advised to take the therapeutic baths; turn to page 159 for instructions.

## STRICT LIVER-CLEANSING DIET LUNCH AND DINNER AT A GLANCE:

### LUNCH AND DINNER: 1 PROTEIN + 2 OR MORE VEGETABLES

- Your protein choice can be meat, poultry, fish, eggs, or lentils/legumes. The general recommendation is a palm-sized serving, though please eat enough to feel satiated.
- Your vegetables can be a mix of starchy vegetables (sweet potato or yam, squash, beets) and plenty of nonstarchy ones (leafy greens, bitter greens, cruciferous, peppers, etc.).
- Use olive oil or flaxseed oil to taste and satiety, salt or seaweed to taste, lemon or apple cider vinegar or a dressing or dip recipe to drizzle—and use plenty of herbs too.

## A NOTE ON EATING DESSERT DURING THE LIVER-CLEANSING DIET

I traditionally do not recommend desserts during cleansing. If dessert is desired, I recommend fresh, poached, grilled, stewed, or baked fruit. Try baked or poached apples or pears with cinnamon, or a fruit compote mixed according to the fruit-combining rules, or a bowl of cherries or fresh berries or peaches if in season. Ideally, wait two hours after eating your meal before eating fruit, to give your digestion a chance to work. A square of 80 to 90 percent dark chocolate can also be used as a sweet treat.

## BLENDED DRINKS

Using a blender to create drinks from vegetables or fruits has some advantages. With blended drinks, we are able to consume more vitamins and minerals from fresh produce than would be possible for the average person to chew. You will find the recipes for my favorite vegetable-based blended drinks on page 216, and I invite you to try them. These can also be of help whenever the digestion is weakened to the extent that raw or even cooked vegetables are hard to digest, or in the case of colitis, as rough salad can create gas and cause inflammation. In these cases, consider drinking blended, cooked vegetables instead of consuming a large bowl of raw salad. When the digestion is weak, steaming vegetables to tenderize them may be enough to help make them digestible, and blending them will make them even easier to digest. You may find this helps if you have a nervous disposition. Often the person who has a sensitive mind also has a sensitive stomach, making raw foods harder to assimilate.

## The Modified Liver-Cleansing Diet: Weeks 4–6

Weeks 4–6 are the Modified Liver-Cleansing Diet, with these simple modifications:

1. You may switch from the Liver-Cleansing Drink at breakfast time to a new breakfast option (such as those listed on page 164) or you may choose to continue the Liver-Cleansing Drink—or alternate between the two. Continue with the same coffee/tea rules.
2. You may add back whole grains (such as rice, millet, barley, farro, amaranth, oats, corn, and whole-grain pasta) and white potatoes. There may be signs that the diges-

## EATING OUT WHILE ON THE PROGRAM

Pick a restaurant where you can order a simply prepared protein and vegetable sides. Often the vegetable sides are listed on the menu separately—in Italian restaurants they are listed as "contorni"—or you may be able to ask for simple steamed sides. Grilled chicken, fish, or meat or lentil soup with vegetables, and the addition of olive oil at the table, would be the ideal. Vegetarian and Indian restaurants will have lentil dishes, either salads or mixed cooked vegetables, and tandoori options. However, keep in mind that most restaurants and delis making prepared foods use poor-quality cooking oils and cook at high temperatures. If you eat out occasionally, it is better not to stress about your food and do the best you can. If you eat out frequently, it might be time to start becoming friends with the chef who is cooking your food so you can ask for what you prefer. Take into consideration that most restaurants use aluminum cooking and baking pans, which will increase your heavy-metal load. It is important to do the Clorox baths to help alleviate this hazard. If your schedule calls for travel, you might not be able to continue drinking the Liver-Cleansing Drink—that is fine; simply follow the Modified Liver-Cleansing Diet while you are on the road by eating half a grapefruit before your breakfast of oatmeal and berries or eggs and vegetables. Just do the best you can!

tion is working better: less white coating on the tongue, improved digestion with less bloat, decreasing sugar cravings, and regular daily bowel movements. If any of the symptoms you noticed before starting are still present, it is suggested to continue on the strict diet, trusting that the body is finding its way toward better digestion. Remember, on the Modified Liver-Cleansing Diet, you will continue to forgo baked goods made from grains, as well as gluten-free baked goods made with tapioca or potato starches.

Please follow the same midmorning/midafternoon snack rules, if desired, as in the strict phase, and at lunch and dinner follow the formatting from the strict phase and adapt it as you like to include the allowed additional foods. Try using the inspiration list on page 164 for ideas. Note that the therapeutic baths are continued during weeks 4–6.

## Therapeutic Baths

The second aspect of the Harmonic Healing program is the therapeutic baths. For over three decades, I have used therapeutic baths to help patients neutralize metals, chemicals, and radiation. These baths are a powerful but gentle and natural alternative to the therapies that are currently popular with those who want to eliminate metals, chemicals, and radiation in their systems. These techniques date back to the early history of naturopathy. Some have even crossed over into the mainstream: The Mayo Clinic recommends a Clorox bath for conditions like eczema. I have found that, when the baths are used regularly, there is a rebalancing at the cellular level. The baths neutralize the metals, chemicals, and radiation in the electromagnetic energy field created in the water of the tub. As the water cools, there is an osmotic exchange of fluids that occurs, and the metals, chemicals, and radiation are released into the bathwater.

These baths use affordable ingredients that can be sourced easily, and they can be done in the convenience of your home. In our era of environmental toxicity, the baths provide an easy way to neutralize these environmental pollutants. I invite you to make the baths a part of your self-care routine. Indeed, it's what my longtime patients tend to love and feel the benefits of the most.

For those without a bathtub, there are many homeopathic combination formulas on the market to neutralize metals. (See "Resources," page 265.) Know that the bombardment is ongoing, so be ready to continue taking the formulas periodically to stay on top of clearing pollution if a bathtub is not available. Infrared saunas are another option, but my preference is to use the baths, for they are easier and cheaper to maintain and offer a much-needed moment for relaxation and restful contemplation.

## Instructions

Baths should be taken in water that is hot, but not so hot that you burn yourself or have a red ring around your butt! Stay in the bath for twenty to thirty minutes or until the water cools down. Those who have high blood pressure or a heart condition should try the baths cooler, in order not to stress the heart. I recommend that you rotate among three different soaks weekly.

Be sure to do the baths one at a time, as they each have a different function, and do not share them with another person. Drink a glass of water during the bath to help move the water in the body and to help detoxification by staying hydrated. If you feel light-headed at any time, carefully get out of the bath or ask for help if needed. It is preferable to avoid showering after the bath, but if you choose to shower, don't use soap. Know that it is quite normal to feel tired after the detoxifying baths, so it is advised to do them before bed so you can rest after the detox.

### CLOROX BATH
(For elimination of chemicals and metallics)

Pour ³/₄ cup of **regular Clorox** into a tub of comfortably tolerable hot water. Soak in the tub for 20–30 minutes or until the water cools. Use only Clorox brand. Do not use scented, powdered bleach, bleach crystals, or any other brand of bleach.

*A note on Clorox. Clorox is a salt. Clorox bleach is made by combining chlorine and caustic soda (sodium hydroxide). Chlorine is bubbled into a solution of water and sodium hydroxide, converting all free chlorine into a solution of sodium hypochlorite. Clorox brand bleach is a 5.25 percent solution of sodium hypochlorite and* water. Because of this, Clorox bleach becomes an oxygenator when diluted into a bath or soak. It is a simple naturopathic treatment of a salt bath with oxygen and it has been used therapeutically for over 75 years.

The Clorox company has not been contacted for consent and is in no way responsible for methods of use other than those listed on the product packaging.

..................

### SEA SALT AND BAKING SODA BATH
(For neutralizing most types of radiation)

Pour 1 pound of pure salt (sea salt or kosher salt—if kosher, check the label to make sure there are no additives) and 1 pound of baking soda into a tub of *comfortably tolerable* hot water. Soak in the tub for 20–30 minutes or until the water cools.

..................

### APPLE CIDER VINEGAR BATH
(For elimination of uric acid deposits and carbon chemicals)

Pour 2–4 cups apple cider vinegar into a tub of *comfortably tolerable* hot water. Soak in the tub for 30 minutes. Sweating sometimes occurs.

Turn to chapter 7 for tips on drinking adequate water, addressing shock, resting well, breathing consciously, and other enhancements to this program that you can do alongside the food and baths if you choose, or that you can use to maintain the program's benefits after you have completed it.

## Homeopathic Alternatives

*Alumina* 30x can be used 3 times daily for 3 weeks. This can be especially useful if you have been eating out a lot or have visited a developing country, which most likely will have exposed you to heavy metals.

*Lycopodium 30c* is a remedy that can also be used to detox aluminum. For general treatment of metallics individually or in combination in the 30x potency, you can use *alumina, plumbum met, mercurius, and arsenicum alb.*

## Putting It All Together

Embarking on a cleansing program takes a little forethought. While there are plenty of delicious foods to eat throughout the six weeks, the way you will feed yourself may be slightly different from your norm, especially if you are used to relying on bread, pasta, rice, potatoes, and so on for much of your intake. If you eat out frequently, you will do best on this program if you choose simple meals at restaurants and begin to consider cooking at home more often or preparing foods in advance if you are on a tight work schedule. If you are accustomed to cooking for your family, introduce them to their new diet of healthy food. And customize a little: Even if you are not eating rice while on the strict diet for the first three weeks, you can make a pot of rice for them or cook a pasta for them to be enjoyed alongside all the beautiful vegetables that you will be eating.

Familiarize yourself with the program by reading through the following section and taking a good look at the pantry section and the recipes starting on page 208.

## INSPIRATION: A WEEK ON THE STRICT PHASE (WEEKS 1–3)

*Below is a sample week of meals for those who eat meat, fish, and eggs. You may of course also choose any of the options from the vegetarian sample menu that do not include grains. If you are on the candida protocol, almost all of the sample meals below will work for you, except that recipes that use vinegar will use lemon juice instead, as noted in chapter 8.*

*Basic instructions are included for many of the below meals. Please note that the menus are designed to bring together the five flavors and tastes to wake up the subtle bodies.*

**NOTE:** *A mug or bowl of Vital Broth (page 217) or Bone Broth (page 220) or blended soup such as Quick Zucchini Soup (page 218) is a warming and digestion-enhancing addition that can be used before any meal.*

| DAY | MENU | |
|---|---|---|
| 1 | BREAKFAST | Liver-Cleansing Drink |
| | LUNCH | Green salad topped with sliced steamed beets and steamed asparagus; 6 oz. poached salmon with a dollop of Aioli *(page 259)*. |
| | DINNER | Sunday Roasted Whole Chicken *(page 251)* and root vegetables with naked steamed spinach |
| 2 | BREAKFAST | Liver-Cleansing Drink |
| | LUNCH | Leftover Sunday Roasted Whole Chicken *(page 251)* on an arugula salad with shaved fennel and radicchio, extra-virgin olive oil, lemon, a few flakes of sea salt, and a twist of black pepper |
| | DINNER | Grilled beef fillet, baked sweet potato, and broccoli rabe steamed with garlic and drizzled with extra-virgin olive oil |

| DAY | MENU | |
|---|---|---|
| 3 | BREAKFAST | Liver-Cleansing Drink |
| | LUNCH | Passato di Verdure *(page 226)* (vegetable soup) with a poached egg added |
| | DINNER | Spiralized Zucchini Noodles with Buffalo or Turkey Bolognese *(page 252)*; steamed escarole drizzled with extra-virgin olive oil |
| 4 | BREAKFAST | Liver-Cleansing Drink |
| | LUNCH | Seasonal vegetable frittata or omelet with spinach and tomato; Boston lettuce salad with finely diced shallots, olive oil, and lemon |
| | DINNER | Grilled lamb chops with baked acorn squash; steamed beets; steamed artichoke with lemon and olive oil or Homemade Mayonnaise *(page 258)* or Aioli *(page 259)* for dipping |
| 5 | BREAKFAST | Liver-Cleansing Drink |
| | LUNCH | Chicken Fajitas *(page 255)* with Calabacitas with Fresh Green Chilies *(page 239)* and Guacamole *(page 262)* |
| | DINNER | Grandma's Chicken Soup *(page 222)* with added escarole |
| 6 | BREAKFAST | Liver-Cleansing Drink |
| | LUNCH | Dr. Linda's Dal with Veggies *(page 230)*; mixed green salad with grated beets, grated carrots, and lemon and olive oil dressing |
| | DINNER | Branzino or other whole or filleted fish with lemon and dill in parchment paper *(instructions provided on page 206)*; steamed bok choy, carrots, scallions, and slivered ginger |
| 7 | BREAKFAST | Liver-Cleansing Drink |
| | LUNCH | Southwest Fiesta Salad *(page 256)* with grilled chicken or beef, with Guacamole *(page 262)* and Salsa Fresca *(page 260)* on the side |
| | DINNER | Dr. Linda's Italian Lentil Soup *(page 223)* and Harmonic Beet Salad *(page 234)* |

*When modifying the Liver-Cleansing Diet to include whole grains, your week could look something like this.*

| DAY | | MENU |
|---|---|---|
| 1 | BREAKFAST | Liver-Cleansing Drink or oatmeal with berries and/or bananas and cream or flaxseed oil |
| | LUNCH | Brown rice with steamed vegetables and shiitake mushrooms |
| | DINNER | Sunday Roasted Whole Chicken *(page 251)* with roasted carrots, white baby potato, and brussels sprouts; endive salad with sliced beets and Simple French Dressing *(page 258)* |
| 2 | BREAKFAST | Liver-Cleansing Drink or vegetable juice, followed by poached eggs over steamed asparagus or other steamed greens |
| | LUNCH | Salad of leftover Sunday Roasted Whole Chicken with Homemade Mayonnaise *(page 251, 258)*, diced red onion, capers, diced carrots, and celery over a bed of Boston lettuce |
| | DINNER | Grilled buffalo burger; Dr. Linda's Coleslaw *(page 253)*; potato salad with grated carrot and Homemade Mayonnaise *(page 258)* |
| 3 | BREAKFAST | Liver-Cleansing Drink or soft-boiled or poached eggs over brown rice vegetable congee, plain congee with vegetables *(see instructions on page 207)*, or brown rice |
| | LUNCH | Sardines over greens with sliced red onion, avocado, lemon, and olive oil |
| | DINNER | Ratatouille *(page 237)* over brown rice or brown rice pasta or with roasted leg of lamb; tri colored salad of endive, arugula, and radicchio with olive oil and lemon dressing |
| 4 | BREAKFAST | Liver-Cleansing Drink or poached, steamed, or slow-scrambled eggs with ghee, with fresh garden greens with apple cider vinegar and olive oil |
| | LUNCH | Quinoa Tabbouleh *(page 240)* and Homemade Hummus *(page 261)* with crudités |
| | DINNER | Grilled marinated or dry-rubbed grass-fed beef fillet with baked sweet potato, steamed asparagus, and steamed beets |

| DAY | MENU | |
|---|---|---|
| 5 | BREAKFAST | Liver-Cleansing Drink or Japanese breakfast: grilled or steamed salmon, rice, and seaweed with fermented vegetables (kimchi), optional |
| | LUNCH | Tomato, eggplant, peppers, onions, and zucchini or frittata or omelet of leftover Ratatouille *(page 237)* with basil; herb salad with mixed greens and lemon and olive oil |
| | DINNER | Grilled Chicken Paillard Salad *(page 244)*; Socca Flatbread *(page 241)* |
| 6 | BREAKFAST | Liver-Cleansing Drink or overnight-soaked muesli with seeds, grated apple, and berries |
| | LUNCH | Passato di Verdure *(page 226)* (green soup) and romaine salad with olive oil and lemon |
| | DINNER | Vegetable Broth *(page 220)*; beef pot roast with onion, carrots, potato, and naked steamed greens |
| 7 | BREAKFAST | Liver-Cleansing Drink or half a fresh papaya with lime, fruit salad, fruit compote, grapefruit, or, in summer, watermelon. |
| | LUNCH | Hard-boiled eggs, poached salmon, capers, grated beets, grated carrot, avocado, lemon, and olive oil on a bed of Boston Lettuce |
| | DINNER | Baked Fish in Parchment Paper *(page 206)*; steamed asparagus with lemon; steamed and mashed turnip/rutabaga drizzled with olive oil and sprinkled with sea salt |

# INSPIRATION: A WEEK ON THE LIVER-CLEANSING DIET FOR VEGETARIANS/VEGANS

All the meals listed below can be eaten for either lunch or dinner. I have two preferred vegetarian meals that are simple and can be varied according to the season:

1. One simply cooked whole grain, one cooked bean, and two or three vegetables steamed, then drizzled with olive oil and a little sea salt (a simple macrobiotic plate)

2. Dal *(see recipe on page 230)* with vegetables of choice, served with basmati rice (optional)

One of these choices per day for lunch or dinner will make your experience simple and straightforward. But you may mix and match your options as you like. Here are some other suggestions to make each day of vegetarian eating on the cleanse varied and fun.

| DAY | | MENU |
|---|---|---|
| 1 | BREAKFAST | Liver-Cleansing Drink |
| | LUNCH | Hummus *(page 261)* with carrot, jicama, and endive; Quinoa Tabbouleh *(page 240)* |
| | DINNER | Baked sweet potato, steamed beets, and steamed artichoke with extra-virgin olive oil dip |
| 2 | BREAKFAST | Liver-Cleansing Drink |
| | LUNCH | Quick Zucchini Soup *(page 218)*, brown rice and steamed vegetables drizzled with olive oil |
| | DINNER | Cuban Black Bean Soup *(page 228)*, Calabacitas with Fresh Green Chilies *(page 239)*, bitter greens salad with olive oil and lemon |
| 3 | BREAKFAST | Liver-Cleansing Drink |
| | LUNCH | Dr. Linda's Kitchari *(page 231)* |
| | DINNER | French Peasant Soup with Pistou *(page 225)* |
| 4 | BREAKFAST | Liver-Cleansing Drink |
| | LUNCH | Grilled Baba Ghanoush *(page 241)* with cucumber and endive leaves, Mediterranean Grilled Vegetables *(page 242)* served with rice and lentils, Jalapeño Sauce *(page 259)* to taste |
| | DINNER | Cannellini Bean and Escarole Soup *(page 227)* with optional whole-grain pasta, arugula salad with lemon and olive oil |

| DAY | MENU | |
|---|---|---|
| 5 | **BREAKFAST** | Liver-Cleansing Drink |
| | **LUNCH** | Dr. Linda's Dal with Veggies *(page 230)*; leafy green salad with lemon and extra-virgin olive oil |
| | **DINNER** | Baked acorn squash with rice or quinoa and herbs, naked spinach |
| 6 | **BREAKFAST** | Liver-Cleansing Drink |
| | **LUNCH** | Bright Yellow Cashew Rice *(page 236)*, Indian-Style Cabbage Bhaji *(page 235)*, grated raw carrots or beet chutney and sliced cucumbers |
| | **DINNER** | Passato di Verdure *(page 226)* with Socca Flatbread *(page 241)* |
| 7 | **BREAKFAST** | Liver-Cleansing Drink |
| | **LUNCH** | Mixed Vegetable Curry *(page 238)* served with basmati rice, millet, or other grain, salad of mixed pungent sprouts with extra virgin olive oil and sea salt flakes |
| | **DINNER** | Carrot-ginger soup, soba noodles with spring vegetables (fresh English peas, asparagus, carrot, and scallion) |

# Troubleshooting During Your Liver Cleanse

Doing the Liver-Cleansing Program helps clear the pathways for the body's healing potential to flow. The following are some of the most common issues that can come up:

- *Constipation:* If the bowels are not moving, the cause can be a lack of bile. Eating adequate beets, apples, and bitter greens, as well as ensuring you are hydrated and drinking the Liver-Cleansing Drink, is helpful.

- *Headaches:* Can occur as toxins move out. The homeo-pathic remedy nux vomica (two 30c pellets dissolved under the tongue three times daily) can often help allevi-ate this symptom.

- *Cravings for sugar or junk food:* These can be helped by put-ting a pinch of sea salt on your tongue or in your drinking water. An alternative is to eat a few olives or sprinkle sea salt flakes on your food.

- *Caffeine cravings:* If you are craving more than one or two cups of caffeine per day, two 30c coffea pellets dissolved under the tongue twice a day can be helpful for a few days or until the craving subsides.

- *Cravings and overindulgence in rich foods:* Nux vomica or carbo vegetabilis can help. Dissolve two 30c pellets of either one under the tongue two or three times daily until cravings and discomfort from overeating subside.

- *Feeling hungry, ungrounded, or spacey:* Be sure to include satisfying portions of root vegetables to ground you and of higher-carbohydrate-content vegetables (yam, sweet potato, squash, beets) with a little sea salt alongside your nonstarchy vegetables, and ensure your quantity of extra-virgin olive oil and flaxseed oil suffices. Sometimes more protein is needed because the blood sugar is low. You may increase to a fourth meal until your blood sugar has balanced.

## Transitioning from the Six-Week Liver-Cleansing Program

Six weeks after starting the Liver-Cleansing Diet and therapeutic baths, you are likely digesting, assimilating, and eliminating better and in general feeling more mentally and emotionally balanced. It is a good time to revisit the list of questions on page 133. Have any of the symptoms that regularly bothered you previously started to abate? Very often, bothersome symptoms have begun to clear up, making it possible to shift from the Liver-Cleansing Diet to what is called the maintenance phase of self-care, in which the basic principles of eating are followed in an ongoing way, with modifications as follows.

If the symptoms that you identified before starting the Liver-Cleansing Diet have not abated, this is typically a sign that another stage of inquiry is warranted. There is another layer to peel back. Revisit chapter 3, "The Five Parasites," and read through the symptoms associated with each one. You may want to consider having your doctor test you for the presence of parasites. If a parasite is detected, you have many options for treatment to discuss with him or her.

The following are the foods you can slowly add back to the maintenance phase after your six-week Liver-Cleansing Program.

### Dairy Products

Milk, yogurt, soft and hard cheeses. Goat-milk products are the easiest to digest. If parasites have been present in the past and have been brought under control during this program, you may well find dairy digestion has improved. If you are sensitive to dairy, you may find that cream in small amounts is well digested because it is a fat and not a protein that can cause irritation in some people. Some people just do not digest dairy well because of their constitution. Dairy can be eaten according to the food-combining rules and not usually more than once a day.

## Nuts and Seeds

Look for raw unroasted nuts and seeds, and enjoy them in small amounts, such as ten to fifteen almonds on a hike with a piece of fruit. A few smears of raw nut butter on apple slices is a good snack. It is best to make nut milks fresh at home if possible, or at the very least look for nut milks with no added cane sugar and minimal additives. Again, do not get in the habit of relying on nuts and nut butters—they are not meal replacements! Soaking nuts and seeds before use can be time intensive but is recommended, as it makes them easier to digest.

Coconut deserves its own mention. While some consider it a type of fruit called a drupe and others call it a nut, my primary concern is that this 100 percent saturated fat is a very heavy fat, so it is to be used in moderation. If there are no palm trees in your neighborhood, then coconut should not be eaten on a daily basis. Coconut oil hardens in colder climates and stays fluid in a hot, tropical climate. This hardening effect can be considered here as a stress to circulation. In evaluating patients who use coconut milk in smoothies, feast on coconut-flour gluten-free baked goods, and use coconut oil for cooking and even eating right off the spoon or in their coffee, I find congestion in their circulation and congested liver and gallbladder. While there are many good things to love about coconuts, especially their antiviral and antibacterial properties, it is wise not to be reliant on coconut oil for these purposes. They also have antiparasitic action: In the years I spent in Sri Lanka, I drank one king coconut daily for its antiparasitic properties, but know that nature provides many herbs with antiparasitic properties from the area you are living in. If you already own a supply of this food, don't despair! A jar of coconut oil is great for slathering on your skin and can continue to be used for your beauty needs.

## Bread and Whole Grains

If you have been avoiding bread and whole grains, you may find that once your liver and bowels are working well, you may begin to digest them in small amounts. If you are eating bread that is made from wheat, it is important to consider the source and to make sure that it is organic. I personally enjoy 100 percent durum organic wheat from Italy. If eating bread causes bloating, consider that the yeast might be more the issue than the wheat. Try sourdough breads, which are made with starter cultures, not with yeast added. If the grains are organic, properly prepared—soaking grains before cooking can reduce their inflammatory potential due to the reduction of plant compounds called lectins—and slow-cooked at a low temperature, you may find you can tolerate them well. Consume bread and whole grains in moderation along with all the other reintroduced foods. If they were prepared with love and made with organic ingredients, then enjoy and savor every bite.

## A Broader Array of Fats and Oils

Try to maintain the principles around fats and oils that you have learned in the Liver-Cleansing Program as often as you can, and know that butter, tallow, and chicken and duck fat can also be included for cooking during the maintenance phase, after the liver is able to digest these good fats again. (Only cook with butter on low heat or add it to vegetables after they are cooked.) I highly recommend avoiding fried foods as an ongoing way of life; this includes French fries, tortilla and potato chips, doughnuts, and of course all kinds of fast food.

Above all, keep your vegetable volume high, enjoying at least four to six servings a day, with an abundance of raw and steamed produce, and remember the options of liquefied vegetable drinks or juices, blended vegetable soups, or vegetables in stews. You will maintain the benefits you gained beautifully, and your body will thank you for it.

A note on alcohol. Too much alcohol can affect the liver detrimentally. The maintenance phase allows spirits and wine in moderation. They have played a part in man's history from ancient times and they serve a purpose. Dr. Parcells used to drink a glass of wine with her dinner most nights. She said it helped her digestion and she enjoyed it! I have known many centenarians in my life, and they did not avoid alcohol but drank it with their meals and in moderation.

The maintenance phase is, in truth, more than a phase; it is a way of life, in which we maintain the benefits we gained on the six-week Liver-Cleansing Program as best we can and also accommodate a greater range of experiences. We want to maintain our new awareness of how foods affect our body and maintain the supportive use of good foods and gentle cooking techniques we have learned as best we can, following the principles outlined during the six weeks in a continuous manner. Yet we also want to allow for the fullness of our lives—we should be able to enjoy eating out, socializing, exploring food culture, and trying new things. In other words, it's about taking care of ourselves in real life! But real life lived with an awareness of the liver and an awareness of energy. In this lifestyle, you may choose to do the Liver-Cleansing Program once or twice a year, as my patients tend to do. You may start to detect when the program is in order—such as when you feel sluggish, tired, or bloated, or if you want to take care of your body after a period of indulgence, overwork, or high demands. You now have the tools to do this—listen to your body, and adopt these tools when it asks.

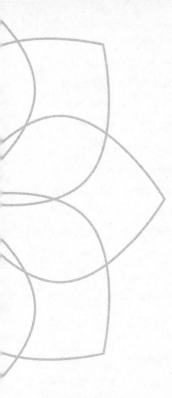

Chapter 7

# Tips for the Liver Cleanse and a Healthy Lifestyle

The following tips are the ones I share with my patients to help them get the most out of their Liver-Cleansing Program and maintain the benefits on a daily basis. They are guidelines that will help to enhance the lifestyle of caring for your liver. You can use this information to improve your experience during the cleanse and continuously to maintain good health.

## Hydration: Honoring Your Body's Need for Water

Patients are asked to drink at least two quarts (eight cups) of water per day. Proper hydration is key to health. Two quarts is a general recommendation; some people may need more and others may need less. Increase water according to your thirst and activity and how much you sweat daily. It is important to drink water to wash your fascia—the web of subtle connective tissue that wraps all your organs, bones, muscles, and nerves, holding you together—and for the lymph to flow.

Adequate intake of water is important. Too little and we become dehydrated, drying up like a prune; too much and we cause stress to the kidneys. Think of it this way: Water is the combination of hydrogen and oxygen (water and air, in element terms): $H_2O$. Water is the third element operating in the body—it is the *kapha* alongside the other two *doshas, vata* (air) and *pitta* (fire). These elements of air, fire, and water work together to create and sustain life in our body. A plant will not live without water, or it will go dry, and without air it will not grow. Without the warmth of fire—or the heat of the sun—there is no color or nourishment to the leaves. We need this balance also—remember, our liver is our "fire" residing in the solar plexus of our body—and the right amount of water helps to keep the fire element in check. I share this information to spark an insight that has gotten lost in our contemporary culture, where many of us drink water all day long—sometimes to excess. Mindful consumption of water matters, but this does not necessarily mean hydrating all day long. It means conscious awareness of our body's need for water in balance.

One thing that is rarely discussed today is that hydration can come from more than just drinking water. It comes from including lots of fresh fruits and vegetables in the diet too, and we are wise to focus on eating them as part of our daily "hydration practice." Fresh fruits or a salad with leafy lettuces, tomato, cucumbers, and celery are hydrating; and plants with a gelatinous substance, such as chia seeds, zucchini, okra, cucumber, and succulents like purslane and aloe vera hydrate especially well. Living in the high desert of New Mexico, where dehydration is a constant possibility, I have learned a great amount about this potential and about conscious intake of water through plant foods.

## Hydration Guidelines

The following rules of thumb will help you hydrate in a manner that gives your body what it needs, without overdoing it or disrupting digestion. If you are toting water during the day, I highly recommend using a glass water bottle or stainless-steel container, not a plastic or aluminum water bottle of any kind, in order to avoid any contamination to the water.

- Drink one, two, or more glasses of room-temperature water on rising.

- Drink one, two, or more glasses of water before and during meals. Stop drinking water for at least two hours after eating to allow your digestion to work. Remember, water is needed for digestion, but in the analogy of the stomach as pot on the stove, when the lid is on the pot and the rice is cooking, we want to avoid lifting the lid and throwing in more water. It will impede the process, as digestion can be interfered with.

- After finishing your meal, a cup of hot water, herbal tea, or water with herbal digestive bitter tonics may be taken, as well as any water required for taking cleansing or detoxifying herbs or supplements.

- You may have a cup of herbal tea before bed if bedtime occurs at least two hours after the meal. It is best not to go immediately to sleep after eating.

- If you work out and sweat during the day, it is important to drink water to replace the loss. (Note: Working out should also occur at least two hours after meals.) And be sure to rehydrate after saunas and during baths.

You may be one of those people who do not feel thirsty or who feel too thirsty. Use a pinch of sea salt in your water and see if that changes how you feel. The salt helps the body absorb the water. I often use natrum muriaticum (homeopathic salt), two 6x pellets taken twice daily for a few weeks, to balance the water in the body.

The body goes through a cycle just as the ocean has tides that ebb and flow. This is called the alkaline tide. At around 3:00–4:00 A.M. and 3:00–4:00 P.M. we dump our toxic wastes and our minerals are at their lowest.

This is why we often feel tired and depleted in midafternoon—the loss of minerals creates a temporarily weakened etheric field. To avoid this, drink water with a pinch of sea salt or squeeze of lemon, or even a fresh vegetable juice to replace the minerals that are lost during this releasing of toxins.

Paying attention to good hydration goes hand in hand with two other essential habits: movement, which moves water around our body, and breathing, for through breath we can absorb the water from the atmosphere, and this also moves our energy. Hydration, movement, and breathing are important parts of the Harmonic Healing lifestyle.

## Movement and Mobility: A Daily Necessity

Although our lives can feel busier than they ever have, much of the busyness takes place sitting down. This is a problem today, because our bodies were meant to move. When we sit still, we become stagnant; our muscles become weak and stiff. As our bodies age, the importance of movement becomes even greater. Sedentary patterns of working at a desk, commuting or driving, and sitting on the couch shorten and weaken the muscles and limit our range of motion. Daily exercise and stretching helps to prevent degeneration and can restore strength, flexibility, and vitality. It also ensures that water moves through our fascia, which plays an important role in transporting hydration into cells, organs, and tissues. Any kind of movement can do this. I recommend starting the day with a short movement program to wake up the body after sleep— stretching every morning for five minutes, to wake the body up and tell it, "Hello" will support mobility, flexibility, hydration to the cells, and energy throughout the body. Twenty to thirty minutes of exercise later in the day further supports hydration and the function of the liver. If you cannot exercise every day, then try not to skip more than one day so that your body gets in this habit. Yoga, tai chi, dancing, walking, swimming, hiking, and biking are all good options. In addition, remember to get up from your chair periodically to move the water. The flow of water in the body has an electrical nature; exercise and movement move water to our cells, helping to charge our electromagnetic energy through the intelligence of the fascia and the etheric field.

## Dr. Linda's Early-Morning Routine

I found yoga in my early twenties and continue to practice asanas today. My personalized morning practice of stretching, done as a start to the day before showering or eating, incorporates simple yoga postures. Try these if you like, moving slowly and with control, avoiding any movement that causes pain and breathing and relaxing into each pose.

- **Both knees to chest (wide to shoulders).** Lying on your back with your feet on the floor, bent knees, and hands holding the backs of the knees, bring your knees toward your chest and allow them to fall wide toward the shoulders. Breathe and relax for twenty to thirty seconds. Rock back and forth along the spine a few times like a baby, allowing the head to be relaxed and come along for the ride.

- **Hamstring "flossing" and lymph draining.** Lying on your back, straighten your legs up to the ceiling. Pump the ankles, driving your heels toward the ceiling three to five times, then bending your knees to relax. Repeat for three sets. In this position I do variations of ankle circles and toe and foot exercises. This is especially good for moving the lymph system.

- **Seated butterfly: sitting up in easy pose with soles of feet together.** With your feet together in butterfly pose (feet drawn toward groin, hands holding feet), gently allow the knees to fall open toward the floor. Feel the groin muscles gently stretch, and if you like, contract and relax the muscles in succession. This pose has helped me maintain long hours seated at my clinic desk.

- **Yoga postures: downward dog and cobra.** To gently open the spine, begin with downward dog, hold for a few breaths, and then gently move into cobra. Repeat for three sets. Try to avoid stress on the shoulders, and hold each position only as long as it is comfortable. To start the day well, I also like to add prayer, giving appreciation for Mother Earth as I look toward the ground in downward dog pose, then thankfulness for the heavens as I look up to Father Sky in cobra pose.

Now we can take our vital awakened body-mind and awakened spiritual connection into yet another day. Always check with your doctor for advice on the best exercise program for you to follow.

## Breathing and the Conscious Breath

There are many types of breathing exercises to rejuvenate and restore; I teach my patients to spend a few minutes each day practicing with the intention of connecting to the breath. My mentor Professor Anton taught us a method of deep and cyclical breathing that has the effect of centering, circulating, energizing, and calming the nervous system. It begins by taking a breath, then bringing awareness to one of our core power centers, called the lower *dantian,* which is the area of the body located below the navel on the front and between the kidneys on the back. This is the center that governs the inspiration of breath. We also bring awareness to our lungs, the center of the body that expires breath. Connecting to these two power centers with intention intensifies the power of the breath.

## PROFESSOR ANTON'S BREATHING EXERCISE

This simple exercise was the first tool we taught our patients while working in the Kalubowila teaching hospital in Colombo, Sri Lanka. Professor Anton knew the importance of oxygen and would describe it thus: "The average person can live without food for about forty days, without water for about four days, and without oxygen for about four minutes." You can see the level of importance each of those vital ingredients to life have, yet we forget that we are even breathing most of the time.

For at least five minutes per day, practice the following breathing exercise. If you prefer, you can also use a practice you already know, such as alternate nostril breathing.

**STEP 1** Start by sitting up straight. Inhale through the nose. Breathing in deeply, filling all lobes of your lungs with air until there is no more room.

**STEP 2** Focusing on the lower power center, the *dantian*, pause at the full point of the inhale; acknowledge the gift that you have given your body.

**STEP 3** Now exhale through the mouth, releasing all possible air. Pause at the complete point of exhale, taking another moment to be conscious of this process.

Continue to repeat slowly.

The process of filling and emptying the lobes of the lungs, along with a pause of acknowledgment, is very simple but can be very powerful. Between the inflow and outflow of the breath we can connect with our sense of oneness. Experiencing those moments consciously is living with more intention and with gratitude—gratitude for the life we have and for the energies of the cosmos, the earth, the food, and the air that nourish us and create peace.

## Rest: Making Sleep a Priority

Sleep habits are more individualized than hydration habits, because everyone's life is different. We all have lists of priorities to juggle because of work, family, and various commitments—and if we're not careful, adequate and good-quality sleep can start to fall low on the list. Ideally, aim to sleep somewhere between seven and eight hours and get to bed as close to 10:00 P.M. as possible. The liver does much of its detoxification work behind the scenes while we are asleep. This is a parasympathetic process, which means that it is best accomplished if we are at rest. So do your best to get to bed early when you are able to do so. When heading into the bedroom, leave all technology outside. Keep the bedroom a place free of TV and Internet and of pinging notifications and middle-of-the-night e-mail checks; your bedroom is best kept as a sanctuary where you can truly restore.

## Dry Brushing: Everyday Lymphatic Support

Dry brushing is a practice that can be used alongside the bath practice and/or especially in times when you do not have access to a bathtub, for it is a very easy and quick way to support the lymphatic system to do its work of cleansing and immune support. Here are the instructions.

Purchase a natural-bristle brush for skin brushing at a health-food store; a similar brush can even be purchased at a hardware store (make sure it has natural bristles, such as a scrub brush used for floors). Every day, before getting into the bath or shower, dry-brush (do not wet-brush) your skin gently, with strokes always going toward the heart. Brush from the feet up the legs to the torso, then brush from the hands up the arms to the neck and chest; and brush gently at the navel, brushing around and up. As you get used to the brushing, you might like to do it a little more vigorously. The process should take less than five minutes to accomplish.

# Addressing Shock: Dissolving Blocks in the Subtle Bodies

These instructions for attending to shock can be used at any time you choose during the Liver-Cleansing Program or during the maintenance phase.

If you have had anxiety, stress, or a traumatic experience such as a divorce or heartbreak, a bankruptcy, a death of a loved one, or an acute injury or illness, you most likely have a level of shock in your subtle field. We do not necessarily need to focus on why the shock is there or why events in the past occurred the way they did; what we want to do is release the shock so that our subtle energy can flow. Simple remedies that anyone can safely use include flower and homeopathic remedies, which can help very gently to release shock and emotional traumas that are blocking your feelings and thoughts. If after reading chapter 2 you feel that you have unresolved shock in your system, or if events occur that create shock—whether major or minor—the following can be used.

Dr. Edward Bach, a renowned homeopath, discovered that flowers in nature have the ability to affect our emotions. How he discovered it is an interesting story, which he shared in his book, *Heal Thyself.* His "Rescue Remedy" mixture was designed specifically to address shock, trauma, crisis, and emergencies. Bach Flower Remedies work in harmony with herbs, homeopathy, and medications and are safe for everyone, including children, pregnant women, and the elderly, as well as pets.

Bach Flower Rescue Remedy, a combination of five flowers including star-of-Bethlehem, can be taken three to four times daily for any current or past shock to the physical, emotional, or mental body. I especially like giving Rescue Remedy to children after injuries because it calms the subtle fields.

There are many books written about homeopathy to explain how the remedies work that you can investigate. The Law of Similars, the Law of Provings, and the Law of the Minimum dose are the basis of homeopathy and take a lifetime to understand. It is energy medicine at the highest level of action. I welcome you to introduce this nontoxic energy medicine to yourself and your family.

## Homeopathic Remedies

Aconite is used frequently for physical, emotional, and mental shock, while arnica is typically used for physical shock due to injury. Take arnica (30c or 200c) for shock after physical injury every two to three hours and continue until the pain subsides and the addition of aconite 30c or 1m for further clearing of the shock from the injury. It is beneficial to partner arnica and aconite because most physical injuries can create shock in the emotional and mental fields too.

Ignatia can be used for deep grief with emotional shock, such as a death in the family, loss of a job or home, divorce, and so on. Dissolve two 200c pellets under the tongue morning and evening as needed for the sadness to be released.

Many different types of bodywork are also beneficial for the clearing of shock, including acupuncture, cranial sacral therapy, reiki, therapeutic touch, feldenkrais, polarity therapy, and gentle Network Spinal Analysis chiropractic. These all support the release of shock and trauma held in the physical body and subtle bodies.

## Mental and Emotional Balance: Finding the Moments

Maintaining emotional balance is very important for balancing health. Meditation and experiencing connection to nature are simple yet potent ways to care for your emotional body.

**Meditation.** There are many methods of meditation that help us to settle in our nervous systems and experience the quiet awareness that lies underneath our busy streams of thought. For some people, prayer is their form of meditation; for others, a yogic or Buddhist technique, or hiking in nature, is their vehicle of choice for getting past the surface of busyness and thought. Meditation techniques are not guaranteed pathways to silence and bliss; they are practices for helping the mind and nervous system learn new habits of slowing and quieting down. When the mind gets quiet, we may be able to experience ourselves as part of the one field of consciousness that is the source of life. Meditation can not only help us discover a new sense of calm that exists within but also help to shift perspective on who we are and why we are here.

I have learned many forms of meditation in my life. One that I recommend frequently to beginners is this simple exercise given by Father Thomas Keating, a renowned Trappist monk and priest who has taught many people how to sit in contemplation, meditation, and prayer through the technique of centering prayer. Father Thomas once said to me, "It is in the intention of sitting down to meditate that God appears." We experience our connection with the divine at the moment our thoughts make the connection or link with the divine.

## FATHER THOMAS KEATING'S SIMPLE MEDITATION

Sit comfortably in a chair or on a pillow on the floor and close your eyes. Inhale and exhale slowly for a few moments, allowing your body to begin to settle. Slow breaths will start the process of slowing your mind. Take as long as you like. Now imagine yourself sitting on the bank of a river. The river is your stream of consciousness. As you sit and breathe slowly, imagine the river moving and flowing too.

Your place on the riverbank is your place of peace, where the only thing you need to do is breathe.

As thoughts appear, and they usually will, observe them on the river, as if they are whispering, "Think me, think me." Or it may be a feeling that comes—boredom, frustration, anxiety, and so on. Watch each feeling too, as it appears on the river. It is as if they are whispering, "Feel me, feel me."

Acknowledge that you're having the feeling or thought. Don't hate it, judge it, critique it, or move against it. But place it in a boat and let it go down the river. Observe it drifting away. Return to your breath. When another thought or feeling arises, welcome it, and then put it in the boat to drift away and return to your peace on the bank of the river.

ı may stay on the peaceful riverbank for as little or as
me as you like. Some days you might have only five min-
, other days you might have more time to relax into the
experience. The effects of this practice include not only settling
the body after stress but also having less reactivity to events
that occur with an increased ability to watch thoughts and feelings from a place of serenity, so that you can respond to outer
circumstances with greater equanimity and clarity.

**Connection to nature.** The quest for health can become so consuming we can forget about one of the simplest remedies of all: connecting
with nature, feeling the earth, holding a tree, observing the clouds in
the sky. Time in nature is restorative to our etheric field and helps us to
ground in our physical bodies. Through our intention to acknowledge
and give thanks to nature, we are reminded that the natural world supports and heals us. This connection can wake up tired senses when we
feel dulled, and it can enliven us to move, play, and enjoy the moment.
We feel refreshed and less anxious when this relationship is nurtured.
Connecting to nature can be as simple as kicking off our shoes in the
park, walking on a beach, taking a walking route to work through a park
with trees and flowers, or filling our home and work space with plants.
Simply stated, nature heals.

## Homeopathic Remedies for Liver and Digestive Issues

Even in the best circumstances, we can experience digestive disturbances
in everyday life. The following homeopathic remedies can be used at
home when the associated symptoms occur—try them in lieu of a medi-
cation you might typically take. They are not intended to treat acute
illness, but are tools in your kit that can help the body find its way to
balance. Doses can be repeated 3 or 4 times, 1 to 4 hours apart. 2 pellets
should suffice for each dose. After giving a remedy, watch and wait in

order to allow the remedy its fullest action. Watch to see i
changing. You may need to go to another remedy if symp

**CARBO VEGETABILIS 6C**—bloating and gas in the stomach, v

**CINCHONA OFFICINALIS 30C**—bloating and foul-smelling gas, sometimes with painless diarrhea.

**LYCOPODIUM 30C**—bloating around the waist and sour belching with a desire for sweet things.

**NATRUM PHOSPHORICUM 30C**—sour taste in the mouth, acid or burning stomach, and a yellow coating on the tongue, or digestive problems after consuming dairy products.

**NUX VOMICA 30C**—for the discomfort associated with eating to excess or overindulgence.

**PULSATILLA 30C**—gastric discomfort caused by eating too much fatty food with bloating, belching and slow digestion.

**SEPIA 30C**—liver sore and painful, flatulence with headache. Sepia is a liver remedy. It acts on the portal system and can be helpful for hot flashes too.

## Food Poisoning (all at 30 c potency):

From fish, fruit, water: *Arsenicum Alb*
From botulism: *Arsenicum Alb*. followed by *Carbo Veg*.
From spoiled food, general: *Nux Vomica*.
From pastry, fat, oil: *Pulsatilla*.

## ınal Note

A healthy lifestyle is not something we master in a day or even a year. We simply grow in our awareness, little by little, and do our best, treating ourselves with kindness at every step. I have also found that when gratitude is the basis of the lifestyle, we take care of our health from the source of subtle energy in small yet powerful ways. For fifty years I have used the Gayatri mantra daily as a prayer for centering and connecting to the subtle and divine energy of life. It is a universal prayer that has guided me and protected me throughout my life.

Gayatri Mantra

> *oṃ bhūr bhuvaḥ svaḥ*
> *tatsaviturvareṇyaṃ*
> *bhargo devasyadhīmahi*
> *dhiyo yo naḥ pracodayāt*

> —Rigveda

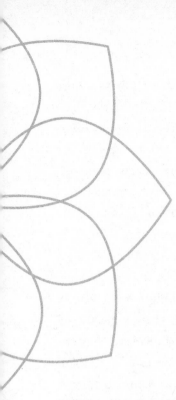

Chapter 8

# Dr. Linda's Kitchen

The kitchen is our studio, where life is created. Cooking can be performed with an artist's sense, a scientist's precision, and a philosopher's deep understanding.

The basic food of life is love. Ideal food is planted with love, watered with love, cultivated with love, harvested with love, and cooked with love. We do the best we can, sourcing good-quality organic, local food, and most important of all, we bless the food. Bless it while you are cooking and bless it when it is on your plate.

When discussing how we should approach shopping, preparing, and cooking on the Harmonic Healing program, I kept coming back to my kitchen. I have had a connection with cooking since I was a child. I learned from my Italian mother, from my Jewish grandmother, and from my studies in Ayurveda and cooking. When I became a mother, the positive effect of high-quality food on my family became obvious. When you have the experience and confidence of cooking for most of your life, combining ingredients and flavors in a harmonious way becomes quite easy, so when I teach my students and patients about food, I try to emphasize that simplicity is best. Complicated combinations are difficult for our digestive systems to process.

I also teach that the process of cooking food imparts a vibration into the food. If we are fearful, stressed, or angry, the food absorbs these energies. Creating a positive relationship with cooking through mindful intention will help to impart a vibration of joy and generosity, and these energies will help to nourish our bodies with the greatest potential. To help limit stress, fear, anger, and frustration in the kitchen, I prepare. Preparation is the key to becoming a successful home cook. In my kitchen pantry and refrigerator, there is usually a bounty of fresh and dry ingredients available that I know I can rely on to make a nutritious meal at home at any time. My style of cooking is what I like to call vegetable forward, with an orientation toward vegetarian food but not exclusively so. I draw from my heritage as well as the many travels I have experienced in my life. As a lifelong student of Ayurveda, homeopathy, and Western and Eastern philosophies, I utilize the medicinal properties of vegetables, spices, and culinary herbs, knowing that food is our first medicine. In our kitchen at Light Harmonics, we incorporate flavors from many cultures that celebrate vegetables, like Mexican/Southwestern cuisine, Mediterranean, and Japanese, and what we may in the United States simply term "farm to table" or "garden to table"—seasonal, sustainable cuisine. We keep a garden in Santa Fe in the spring through fall months, and we try to eat something from the garden every day, even if only herbs. Drawing from these many different flavor profiles, cooking becomes exciting for everyone involved. My kids always looked forward to Southwest fiesta night or pasta night, and I did too, removing the tortilla and cheese if I was cleansing my liver, or making a fajita salad or using zucchini spirals with homemade sauce instead of pasta. These are examples of how you can modify meals to stay within the guidelines of the cleansing program. No matter what foods we remove during a cleanse, we try to create an atmosphere of abundance, gratefulness, and joy in the kitchen. Over my many years of cooking, I have never lost my gratitude for being at the sink or stove.

What follows are some basic tips to get you started on the path of cooking during a Liver–Cleansing Program and creating health through your daily choices in the kitchen. Listed are staples from my dry and fresh pantry, cooking equipment, and instructions for basic cooking methods, with recipes from my years of experience both as a chef and as a home cook for meats, poultry, chicken, eggs, vegetables, legumes, grains, soups, and dressings.

When making meals from scratch and not out of a can or prepackaged, some advance planning is needed. For example, if you are going to create a Southwest fiesta and you want to serve black beans, those beans have to be soaked starting the day before.

Before we go shopping, let's first assess your current kitchen.

**Identify unhealthy ingredients lurking in your kitchen.**

Gather any processed foods or containers with food labels that show added sugar and other ingredients.

**Carefully read labels . . . then toss the junk!**

Ideally, you have already tossed any packaged foods with unhealthy ingredients, but sometimes you have to look a bit closer. If you decide to keep any packaged foods with labels, here are some tips.

Focus on the ingredient list; if you don't recognize a word, you can't pronounce it, or it looks like it's in Latin, then don't use it. The most abundant ingredients are listed first, and the rest are in descending order by weight. If there is a health claim like "no sugar" or "diet" on the label, beware, because this may just be a marketing ploy and sweeteners may be hidden in other ingredients that you may not be familiar with. It will be much easier to focus on cleansing your body when your kitchen has first been detoxified.

Now we can focus on what to put in your kitchen.

# Dr. Linda's Pantry

## Seasonal Fruits and Vegetables

When shopping for fruit and vegetables in your local store or farmer's market, follow these basic tips.

**Seasonal:** Where do you live? What season is it? You shouldn't buy watermelons or tomatoes in the winter in Wisconsin. See more on page 118 for guidance on purchasing seasonal produce.

**Location:** Where was the produce grown? Did it have to travel a long distance to get to you? The longer it had to travel, the less likely you should buy it, because food loses vitality the older it gets.

**Quality:** Check if your produce is organic. The easy check is to look at the number on the label, if it's purchased at a supermarket. If it's a four-digit number, the produce is not organic. If the number begins with a 9 and is more than four digits, it is certified organic. If your food has been conventionally grown, use the Clorox Food Bath on page 144 to clean it.

**Use your senses:** Look at, smell, and touch produce to identify characteristics of high energized food. Choose colorful, vibrant, ripened produce that will energize you and your family for the coming week. Fresh, local produce will typically last days longer than store-bought that has traveled long distances. There is an etheric energy and vitality in produce that you may sense.

The following ingredients are the backbone to creating healthy and delicious meals from the kitchen.

## Citrus (Lemon, Lime, Grapefruit, Orange)

I usually have grapefruit, lemons, and limes—all high in vitamin C and fiber—on hand to use in cooking, dressings, and beverages. Because of its astringent, sour nature, citrus benefits the liver, cleanses the blood, improves circulation, improves mineral absorption, is antiseptic, is antimicrobial, and thins mucus. It is especially effective for colds, flus, coughs, dysentery, and even parasitic infestation. Lemon and grapefruit are key ingredients in the Liver-Cleansing Drink. Orange can also be used in the Liver-Cleansing Drink as a substitute for grapefruit.

## Fresh Berries (Blueberry, Raspberry, Strawberry)

Rich in vitamins B, C, and K and minerals, berries tend to be both sweet and sour, benefiting the liver, kidneys, spleen, pancreas, and blood. When in season, fresh wild berries are some of nature's best antioxidant gifts.

## Apples

Rich in vitamins A, $B_1$, $B_2$, $B_6$, and C, as well as folate and potassium, apples are both sweet and sour, aiding in moistening the lungs and cleansing the liver and gallbladder. Their malic and tartaric acids help to soften gallstones, and their pectin helps to resolve unhealthy cholesterol, heavy metals, and even radiation.

## Avocados

Avocados are a good source of vitamins C, $B_6$, E, and K, folate, magnesium, niacin, pantothenic acid, potassium, riboflavin, and lecithin. They are cooling and sweet, are lubricating and healing to the lungs and intestines, support brain function, and are an easily digested good fat.

*The Holy Trinity:* carrots, celery, and onions. I start many dishes, soups, and stews with these three ingredients. As they are available year-round, it is rare that I do not have them in my refrigerator.

## Carrots

A good source of vitamins A (from beta-carotene), $B_6$, and K, biotin, and potassium, orange and sweet, carrots benefit the lungs, liver, spleen, and pancreas. They stimulate elimination, are diuretic, and help to dissolve accumulations like stones or tumors. Carrots also contain an essential oil that destroys pinworms and roundworms.

## Celery

High in antioxidants, enzymes, vitamins $B_6$, C, and K, folate, and potassium; cool in nature; green, sweet, and bitter; celery benefits the stomach, spleen, and pancreas and calms the liver. It purifies the blood, calms nervousness and vertigo, and calms excess-heat conditions like burning in the eyes and urine, acne, and canker sores. Because of the fibrous quality of celery, it creates a feeling of fullness after eating and can be used for appetite control. It is also one of the few vegetables that can be combined with fruit.

## The Onion Family (Onion, Garlic, Leek, Chive, Scallion)

High in vitamin C, fiber, folic acid, calcium, iron, and quercetin, onions are pungent and support the lungs. Onion is rich in sulfur, which helps to purify the blood, extinguish parasites and heavy metals, and metabolize amino acids. Onions pair well with animal protein.

## Tomatoes

A summertime favorite, vine-ripened fresh heirloom tomatoes are best. Tomato is high in fiber, vitamins A, $B_6$, C, K, and E, thiamine, niacin, folate, magnesium, phosphorus, copper, potassium, and manganese. Cooling, sweet, and sour in flavor, tomatoes benefit the stomach, cleanse the liver, and calm heat in the liver. Thus they can calm hypertension, red eyes, and even headaches. Caution: Tomato is in the nightshade family and can interrupt calcium metabolism. If you have joint pain, arthritis, tendonitis, or other chronic musculoskeletal pain, it is best to limit or avoid tomatoes in your diet. Cooking can reduce toxicity.

## Cucumbers

Cucumbers are high in vitamin K, chlorophyll, and molybdenum, as well as copper, potassium, manganese, magnesium, biotin, and vitamins

$B_1$ and C. Because of their high amount of molybdenum, look to cucumbers when cleansing candida. Cool and sweet, cucumbers are a diuretic, help to clean blood, and support the heart, spleen, pancreas, stomach, intestines, and lungs. Because of their cooling and moistening property, cucumbers are helpful during inflammatory or heat conditions.

## Lettuce

There are many lettuces to choose from. When possible, I prefer to grow and pick my own. When shopping, it is best to look for the freshest leaves and simply choose what you like. Personally, I love all lettuces, from soft butter lettuces to crunchy romaine. Rich in fiber, chlorophyll, vitamins $B_1$, $B_2$, $B_6$, and C, manganese, magnesium, potassium, calcium, chromium, phosphorus, copper, and iron, lettuce is cool, bitter, and sweet. It can be used as a diuretic to help with edema. Lettuce is one of the few vegetables that can combine with fruit.

## Bitter Greens

Similar to lettuce, I look for what is fresh either in my garden or at the local food co-op. I love bitter leafy greens like arugula, escarole, broccoli rabe, Swiss chard, beet greens, chicory, dandelion, frisee, and mustard greens. Rich in many vitamins and minerals, bitter greens have a cleansing effect on the liver and blood. We eat bitter greens regularly in our house.

## Beets

One of my truly favorite root vegetables, beets are almost always in my refrigerator already steamed or ready to cook. They are rich in fiber, vitamin C, folate, potassium, and manganese, as well as phytonutrients that help to ward off cancer. Beets support energy and stamina, support the immune system, and regulate inflammation. Because of their high nitric oxide content, beets lower blood pressure, while the betaine pigments support the body's detoxification process. Beets strengthen the heart, purify the blood, and benefit the liver. Beets are a source of betaine, which helps protect the cells from environmental stress.

## A NOTE ON KALE

Raw kale has lately become something of a superfood. Kale is full of vitamins and minerals and is a phytoestrogen. It is also possibly goitrogenic (similar to broccoli), which means one must be cautious about overeating raw kale if one's thyroid is known to be low (hypothyroidism), because this food can inhibit the body's ability to utilize iodine. The thyroid absorbs iodine from food and combines it with the amino acid tyrosine to create the thyroid hormones T-4 and T-3. Thyroid hormones circulate through the blood as needed to control metabolism, converting oxygen and calories to usable energy. When there is a lack of iodine-rich foods in the diet in combination with absorption inhibition, symptoms associated with hypothyroidism can manifest, such as feeling cold, weight gain, lassitude, and fatigue. Steamed kale, as well as steamed broccoli, is better than raw in these cases. Seaweeds can also be added to the diet to balance the thyroid. (Interestingly, Japanese cuisine includes a large amount of broccoli, cabbage, and soy, which all inhibit iodine absorption, but this is balanced by plenty of iodine-rich seaweed.) Eating too much of any ingredient, even if it is a "superfood," is generally not a good idea. Varying your vegetables daily and eating all parts of the whole plant is the best choice for health.

## Sweet Potatoes

Sweet potatoes contain water, fiber, and important nutrients such as vitamins A and C, manganese, and other vitamins and minerals needed for growth. They store easily in the refrigerator and are simple to prepare, whether steamed, baked, grilled, roasted, or simmered in soups and curries. With the many varieties available in today's market, they are truly a delicious and convenient health food.

## Sprouts

Sprouts are wonderful for their nourishing and building qualities. Avoid alfalfa sprouts due to their susceptibility to mold; if you do use them, store them in the fridge with a paper towel around them to avoid moisture buildup.

## Oils and Dry Goods

The following ingredients can be purchased at your local health-food store or supermarket. If possible, buy in bulk to avoid excess packaging and plastics.

Ghee: Also known as purified butter, ghee helps release spices during cooking and stimulates the digestive fire. Ghee may also be spooned onto rice or a chapati when the meal is served. Because ghee is purified by cooking, it does not become rancid.

Grass-fed sweet butter (unsalted): This may be used during the maintenance phase.

Extra-virgin olive oil: Select oil from the first cold press.

Grapeseed oil: This may be used for cooking.

Sesame oil: This may also be used for cooking.

Flax oil: Use this raw.

Ground flaxseed: This is one of our greatest sources of omega-3 fatty acids. Omega-3s are needed to help regulate inflammation, regulate the bowels, and strengthen immunity. Ground flaxseed is used in the Liver-Cleansing Drink.

Tahini: This is a good source of calcium.

Quinoa

Short-grain and long-grain brown rice, basmati rice, white and brown

Various dried lentils and legumes

Umbrian Italian lentils, French green lentils, red and yellow lentils (dal), chickpeas, black beans, Tuscan white beans, mung beans, adzuki beans, kidney beans

Wheat-free tamari

Organic apple cider vinegar

Glass-jarred tuna, anchovies, sardines (packed in olive oil, spring water, or escabeche)

Glass-jarred tomato paste and whole tomatoes

*Please note:* If you are using packaged, cooked beans or fish, purchase glass jars and not cans to avoid metal, when possible and if available. It is becoming more common for health-food stores and supermarkets to offer glass-jarred fish and beans. Fresh fish and dried beans are preferable, though.

# Herbs, Spices, and Seasonings

**High-quality sea salt (Maldon, Hawaiian, Celtic, or Italian/French):** It is important to pick salts that have no artificial ingredients added and have not been stripped of their naturally occurring essential minerals and electrolytes. The body can assimilate these salts more easily and avoid the unwanted side effects of eating too much table salt, like high blood pressure and dehydration.

**Vegetable salts (herbamare or spike):** Vegetable salts are an enjoyable replacement for table salt that are typically combined with assorted vegetable powders and seasonings.

**Seaweed (dulse flakes, wakame, hijiki):** Seaweed is anticoagulant and antiviral, benefits the thyroid, and is rich in vitamins and minerals including iodine, iron, and vitamins $B_{12}$, C, and K, as well as fiber. Seaweed is a key ingredient used in macrobiotic and Japanese diets along with fish and vegetables. A small amount of seaweed added to soups, rice, and salads packs a large amount of beneficial nutrients.

**Freshly ground black pepper:** Black pepper is anti-inflammatory, supports detoxification, is antioxidant, promotes intestinal health, and is high in manganese, vitamin K, iron, zinc, potassium, and fiber. Whole peppercorns ground fresh as needed are preferable in order to reduce toxicity.

**Cayenne pepper (ground):** Cayenne helps circulation, promotes the healing of ulcers and sores, supports detoxification, is high in vitamins A and C, and is antifungal and antibacterial.

**Basil (fresh or dried):** Basil is anti-inflammatory and high in antioxidants.

**Oregano (fresh, dried, or oil):** Oregano is antibacterial, antifungal, high in antioxidants, and antiparasitic.

**Marjoram (fresh or dried):** Marjoram aids in digestion, has sedative properties, and is antispasmodic.

**Thyme (fresh or dried):** Thyme can thwart intestinal worms, gastrointestinal symptoms, lack of appetite, and anemia, and it is antifungal.

**Cilantro (fresh leaves) and coriander (ground seeds):** Both from the same plant, also called Chinese parsley, these are great heavy-metal cleansers. It is commonly used with pungent and spicy dishes like Indian curries and Mexican salsas. Before use, the leaves and tender upper stalks should be washed and roughly chopped. The oils present in coriander seeds help to assimilate starchy foods and root vegetables and have a cooling effect after digestion.

**Rosemary (fresh or dried):** Rosemary is a tonic, astringent, carminative, and soothing to the nerves.

**Chilies (fresh or dried):** Spicy and warming, chilies strengthen circulation and are high in vitamins A and C.

**Garlic (fresh):** High in manganese, vitamins $B_1$, $B_6$, and C, selenium, calcium, copper, potassium, phosphorus, and iron, garlic reduces heart disease and is a natural antibiotic, antiviral, antifungal, and antiparasitic.

**Bay leaves (dried):** High in vitamins A and C and folic acid, bay leaves help regulate body metabolism.

**Mint (fresh or dried):** Mint is an antiflatulent, aids in digestion, treats colic, colds, and flu, and relieves pain.

**Parsley (fresh, flat-leaf):** Packed full of vitamins A, $B_6$, C, K, thiamine, riboflavin, niacin, pantothenic acid, folate, calcium, copper, iron, magnesium, manganese, phosphorus, potassium and zinc, parsley is also high in chlorophyll and is a natural breath freshener. It is a digestive aid and supports the kidneys and bladder—throughout history, parsley tea has been used for kidney stones and bladder infections.

**Ginger:** Whether fresh or dried, ginger is a good source of vitamins $B_6$ and $B_5$, potassium, manganese, copper, and magnesium. It induces sweating, stimulates the digestive fire, neutralizes toxins, combats nausea, and aids the absorption of food in the intestines. It is always advisable to have some ginger in the kitchen.

**Black mustard (rai) seeds:** Their taste is pungent and nutty. These seeds are used in every fodni and dal. They develop their aroma and flavor when added to hot ghee and allowed to pop and split open.

**Asafoetida (hing) powder:** This aromatic resin comes from the root of the plant *Ferula asafoetida* and is used in small amounts for its distinctive taste and medicinal properties. It helps to prevent flatulence and aids digestion.

**Cumin (jeera):** Cumin not only flavors food but also has many medicinal properties. It can be useful in the treatment of female urinary disorders, problems with the uterus, and excessive white vaginal discharge and is valuable in combating urinary infections, dysentery, gas, and stomach problems. Jeera can also restore the sense of taste. To gain the best medicinal effect, it is recommended that one teaspoon be soaked overnight and the water drunk the next morning. As a kitchen spice, jeera should, like mustard seeds, be cooked in ghee until the seeds become light brown and develop their distinctive aroma.

**Kadi patta (curry) leaves:** Kadi patta leaves are the Indian counterpart to the European bay leaves. They are used to help digestion. When cooked with vegetables and dal (lentils), kadi patta leaves give fragrance and taste. Medicinally, they can be used in the case of dysentery, as a tea to stop vomiting, and against fever.

**Turmeric (haldi):** Turmeric is used in small amounts to give a warm, pungent flavor to vegetables and soups, or simply added to rice dishes. Turmeric helps circulation and purifies the blood.

**Red chili powder:** The powder is made from dried red chilies. Chili stokes the digestive fire, causes sweating, and enhances the taste of the food. It is high in vitamins A and C and increases circulation.

## Kitchen Equipment

Basic equipment: In my kitchen, I use heavy-gauge stainless-steel pots. When I was eighteen, a salesman came to the house and demonstrated waterless stainless cookware, which creates a seal or vacuum that cooks the food in its own juices, and I was so impressed, I purchased them on a monthly plan. At that time, it was a big investment for me. I still use those same waterless, heavy-gauge stainless-steel pots today—when we invest in quality, the price will pay for itself. Any kind of heavy gauge stainless-steel pots will do, although I love a waterless stainless steel pot the best. If it is a good quality stainless steel, a magnet sticks to the pot easily. In addition, I use enamel-covered cast-iron cookware; my mother relied on a collection of pots from Europe, and I still use the very same ones today. (Similar ones are readily available from brands such as Le Creuset and Staub.) You don't need a plethora of different items to cook well; in fact, you can cook most of my recipes with a large Dutch oven. The following key kitchen equipment items are what I recommend (note that you should avoid using aluminum cookware, aluminum foil, and nonstick cookware—they all have the potential to be toxic):

One medium and one large enamel-covered cast-iron Dutch oven

Cast-iron skillet

Grill pan (if you do not have access to an outside grill)

Large (six- to eight-quart) heavy-gauge stainless-steel pot

One large heavy-gauge stainless-steel skillet with cover

Stainless-steel stock pot

Roasting pan (stainless-steel, enamel-covered cast iron, or glass)

Stainless-steel steaming basket

Nonbleached parchment paper

Stainless-steel or wood cooking utensils (avoid plastic)

A good-quality blender (Vitamix is the crème de la crème, but any good blender will do)

## Dr. Linda's Cooking 101

There are many delicious ways to cook proteins and vegetables using little or no cooked oils during a cleansing period of restoring the liver. Steaming, poaching, baking, roasting, grilling, braising, simmering, sautéing in water or broth, and blending are easy to do and require minimal know-how. The following basic instructions will help you put together meals from good ingredients without having to follow complex recipes. Use them during your program—and afterward, for they form an approach to cooking that supports healthy liver function year-round. I prefer to keep it simple in the kitchen to let the ingredients shine. I have taught my children and students these same basic techniques, which are the backbone of my clean cooking and eating program. Once you master them, you can mix and match vegetables and proteins, allowing your inner creative chef to come out. For example, my son often prepares fresh and healthy lunches for us at the office. In the summertime, he will check the garden to see what is ready to pick, then combine it with what staples we have available in my refrigerator and pantry. He might make a zucchini, broccoli, carrot, and onion water stir-fry with wheat-free tamari and poached egg; grilled chicken thigh with steamed Swiss chard and beets; or a fresh-picked lettuce salad with cucumber, radishes, radish greens, basil, tomatoes, and jarred Mediterranean tuna. Our meals are always healthy and delicious, but their content depends on what we have fresh and available. When you do not have access to a garden, it takes a bit more planning to make sure you have your staples available in the kitchen. Regardless of what ingredients are available, have fun and keep it simple. Use the principles.

## FIVE SIMPLE TIPS FOR VEGETABLE COOKING

1. Add slivers of garlic when steaming bitter greens.

2. Try to avoid steaming frozen vegetables except for freezer staples like frozen peas, which are helpful to have on hand for curries. Frozen vegetables have been partially cooked and hence retain less of their life-force value and flavor. If there is no other choice, frozen organic vegetables are better than no vegetables and can be included if needed.

3. Steam asparagus whole. My mother taught me to break off the ends of the tough stem by finding the spot where it "snaps" most easily, about one inch from the bottom. Steam in a pan in a little water, cover and simmer for 10 minutes. Asparagus spears are always so beautiful on the plate.

4. Artichokes can be steamed whole, either in a steamer basket or in a pot with water until tender. They take at least 30 minutes—often longer for tougher ones. Artichokes are especially festive when served on a beautiful ceramic plate with olive oil or Aioli (page 259) to dip. Even small children can enjoy the adventure of tackling the artichoke (cut off the tips of the leaves with scissors before cooking if they are sharp ones). Served with a baked sweet potato, sliced steamed beets, and bitter greens such as broccoli rabe, and generous drizzles of olive oil, artichokes are the star of the meal!

5. Two good everyday steamed vegetables are green beans (stems snipped off, cut into uniform lengths or left whole) and carrots cut into one-inch chunks. Both add color and nutrition and are easy to pair with almost all other vegetables.

## Easy Steamed Vegetables

Steaming is one of the simplest ways to cook vegetables. Herbs and citrus can be used to infuse flavor easily. I like to finish steamed vegetables with extra-virgin olive oil, lemon, and sea salt flakes and fresh ground pepper to taste. It is quick, easy, and delicious!

Vegetables can be easily steamed in a stainless-steel steamer. Check for tenderness after 10–15 minutes (5 minutes for spinach).

Alternatively, use this method, which steams vegetables in their juices. Wash vegetables. Place in heavy stainless steel or enamel cast iron pot, add $^{1}/_{2}$–1 inch of water, cover, and simmer covered on low heat. Most leafy greens will take 5-8 minutes, and heartier vegetables can take 10–20 minutes. You can check after 5 minutes to see if more water is needed (usually not) and to check tenderness. After you get used to cooking this way, it becomes natural. Don't add excessive water; the vegetables will release water, allowing them to "cook in their own juices" to bring out their flavor. Timing is everything if you are steaming vegetables to be served hot with your meal. Knowing how long your sweet potato will take will help you to know when to start your vegetables 10–15 minutes before it's done. A sweet potato that has been cut into chunks will typically take about 20–30 minutes, depending on the size of the pieces. For a faster cook time, you can cut the potato into smaller pieces.

## Simple Steamed Beets

I recommend eating beets weekly and ideally three times a week on a Liver-Cleansing Program, because their beta pigments support the detoxification process, help with elimination through the bowels, and purify the blood and liver. Luckily, they are available year-round—for eons people stored them in the root cellar to nourish themselves through the seasons. I prefer deep crimson beets, but yellow and orange ones make for nice variety. Make beets a staple of your diet. They can easily be grated raw onto any salad.

Place washed, unpeeled beets in a steamer or in a cast-iron pot with water halfway up the tops of the beets, and simmer for about 30 minutes.

Check for tenderness: If a fork pierces the beet easily, take off heat; if not, continue cooking for 5–10 minutes and check again. If desired, add the beet greens on top of the cooking beets at this 30-minute mark and steam until the greens are tender, 10–15 minutes. Put beet greens aside to be used in other dishes. Run cold water over cooked beets, slipping the beet skin off by rubbing with your fingers—they will get a bit red but the stain will wash off. Serve beets any way you like: hot, "naked" (no oil), or with a drizzle of olive oil and a pinch of sea salt. Or chill for later use. Having these in the refrigerator allows you to easily slice onto a salad throughout the week for lunches or use in the Harmonic Beet Salad, page 234.

## Simply Poached Proteins

### Poached Chicken

Pour a few inches of water into a heavy-bottomed pot with herbs such as dill and parsley, and white wine if desired, and bring to a simmer with the lid on. Add 2 split boneless chicken breasts, and, if desired, vegetables such as bok choy, scallions, and carrots. Place in pot and let simmer for 15–20 minutes. Check to see if vegetables are tender and if chicken pulls apart easily—if so, it is done. Try serving with a little of the cooking broth and a dollop of Homemade Mayonnaise (page 258) or Aioli (page 259). You can also use this method for fish or follow the Poached Fish Fillets recipe on page 257.

### Poached Eggs

Heat 3–4 inches of water in a saucepan, add a splash of apple cider vinegar or lemon juice, bring water to a boil, then turn down the heat to simmer. Crack an egg into a bowl, then, using a spoon, stir the simmering water to create a "whirlpool" and drop egg into the middle of it. Let cook until whites are set. If you prefer a runny yolk, this will take about 3 minutes; for a set yolk, about 5 minutes.

## Baked and Roasted Vegetables

Baked sweet potatoes, yams, and squashes can be the center of a simple meal when cleansing, served with steamed vegetables. Cook several at a time and store extras in the refrigerator if you like.

Preheat oven to 375°F. Poke washed sweet potatoes or yams several times with a fork. Place directly on oven rack for 45 minutes–1 hour or until a fork easily pierces the skin.

For squash (acorn squash, butternut, etc.), cut squash in half, remove seeds, poke with a fork, and place in a roasting pan, cut side down, with 1 inch of water. Bake for 30–45 minutes or until a fork easily pierces the skin.

## Braised Meat, Poultry, and Fish

Braising is a great technique for cooking meat, poultry, or fish without oil. Use a heavy iron skillet or enameled cast-iron pot with lid (a braiser). Place a small piece of parchment paper in bottom of pan and set on stove with heat at medium-high. When paper begins to turn brown, place meat, poultry, or fish in the pan to be seared. Turn over when it is browned and releases from pan easily. When both sides are seared, add a cup or so of finely chopped celery, carrots, onions, or garlic, sun-dried tomatoes, and olives. Any desired seasoning combination can be used, such as rosemary and thyme, depending on how you feel. Now you need to add a liquid to braise the meat. You can use white or red wine or even apple cider vinegar, with an equal amount of water. Do not cover the meat; halfway up the meat usually works. Put the heavy lid on and cook on low heat for 2–3 hours. Beef requires more time than chicken.

## Grilling

There is no need to oil the meat if the grill or grill pan is hot enough to sear it. There is enough natural fat in most meats to dry-grill: Place meat, chicken, or fish (skin side down) on hot grill pan and turn when meat lifts easily from grill, usually around 8–10 minutes. You don't need any herbs or flavors to grill meat if you don't have the time. Or you can try the Southwest Dry Rub (page 254). I suggest grilling a few chicken breasts at once and storing extras in the refrigerator to use on salads for the next two or three days.

## Baked Fish in Parchment Paper

Baking in unbleached parchment paper is a clean way of cooking fish using steam that builds up inside. The herb-covered fish looks pretty when unwrapped—and involves minimal cleanup.

Place fish fillet on parchment paper and season with sea salt, black pepper, and one or two fresh herbs of your choice, such as basil, rosemary, thyme, parsley, or cilantro. Add dashes of added flavor if you like—play with paprika, sundried tomatoes, and olives. A tiny drizzle of olive oil for flavor can be used here. Top with slices of lemon. You can add zucchini, yellow squash, baby tomato, onions, garlic, etc. It just depends on what season it is or what your mood is.

Fold the paper all around the fish, crimping the edges tightly so the steam will stay in. Bake at 375°F for 10–20 minutes. You will smell a delicious aroma of the fish cooking. Open package, transfer fish to plate, and drizzle with extra-virgin olive oil, or serve fillets in their pockets and let each guest open their own when everyone is at the table.

## One-Pot Meals

When we think of one-pot meals, we think of winter and slow-cooker meals like stews, ragouts, chili, and vegetarian rice and bean dishes. However, one-pot meals can be cooked and enjoyed all year-round, and they involve minimal cleanup. Below are the simplest instructions for creating a tasty one-pot meal.

If you are using a meat protein, such as a pot roast, sear according to the braising instructions on page 205. This helps render the fat off the meat to create a good flavor base. When protein is seared, with a brown crust, set it aside, add a sliced onion to the pan, and cook on low heat for

10 minutes or until onions are translucent and developing a base layer of flavor. Add celery, carrots, broccoli, turnips, or any other hearty vegetables, such as winter squash, cut into chunks. Quantities of each ingredient can be determined based on what you have on hand and are in the mood for. (This is a rustic dish—no need to finely dice.) Meanwhile, add spices or herbs of your choice—if you're not sure, use a pinch of thyme, rosemary, or herbes de Provence and season with sea salt and pepper to taste. Add 2–2$^{1}/_{2}$ cups of broth or other liquid, such as red or white wine. Bring to a simmer, return meat to pan, cover, and let cook with the vegetables until meat is tender, approximately 2–3 hours.

## One-Pot Grain Bowl

Rice or other grains can be cooked in a heavy cast-iron pan as a one-pot grain meal with or without beans, by adding vegetables such as the "holy trinity" while cooking, then adding cooked beans in the last 10 minutes of cooking and serving with slices of avocado, radishes, or fresh herbs. A dish called congee—simple rice porridge—is recommended for sensitive stomachs and can be served as a meal: Rinse 1 cup brown rice, drain, and place in pot. Add 5–6 cups water or vegetable stock, $^{1}/_{2}$ teaspoon sea salt, and a one-inch knob of ginger, peeled and sliced thin. Stir in any vegetable you may have on hand, such as green squash, broccoli, green beans, kombu (seaweed), spinach, or carrots, cut into small pieces. Bring to a boil, then simmer for at least an hour, stirring every 15 minutes or so. Add more water as needed. This is a loose porridge with vegetables. Check for tenderness of vegetables. Serve with sliced scallion or cilantro or dulse flakes. This is a creamy dish and soothing to the digestive system. I have recommended congee to many patients over the years who were recovering from IBS (irritable bowel syndrome).

One-Pot Grain Meals can then be served in one bowl and garnished with scallions, fresh herbs, or a even a spoonful of Aioli (page 259) or Homemade Mayonnaise (page 258), or drizzled with extra-virgin olive oil.

# No-Fry Stir-Fry Vegetables

Traditional Japanese stir-frying usually fries with sesame oil. However, we try not to fry foods on a liver cleanse. While an occasional sesame oil stir-fry is usually tolerable throughout the program and in the maintenance phase (sesame can tolerate heat), the following oil-free method lets you fill your bowl with vegetables easily, no frying required.

## STEP 1: PICK YOUR VEGETABLES

### GOOD COMBINATIONS

Broccoli, carrots, mushrooms, and Swiss chard

Cauliflower, carrot sticks, and snow peas

Asparagus, shiitake mushrooms, and fresh water chestnuts

Green beans, red peppers, and cremini mushrooms

Potatoes, eggplant cubes, diced green peppers, and cilantro

Bok choy, carrots, scallions, and ginger

## STEP 2: FOLLOW THESE INSTRUCTIONS

1. Cut up vegetables before starting to cook.
2. Heat skillet or wok over medium flame.
3. Pour in 3 tablespoons chicken or vegetable broth.
4. Stir-fry onion, mashed garlic, fresh ginger, or chilies for 2 minutes.
5. Add hard-textured vegetables. Stir, then place cover on skillet and steam 10 minutes.
6. Add softer vegetables.
7. Be careful not to overcook. Cooked vegetables should be tender but not limp.
8. Add a splash of sherry or rice vinegar or wheat-free tamari, if desired.

**STEP 3: TAKE IT FURTHER (IF YOU LIKE)**

To enhance the dish, you can add to the above any of the following steps:

Add mung bean threads—soak first and add as the last ingredient.

Stir in 1–2 eggs at end of cooking and slowly cook, stirring, until they are scrambled.

Add arrowroot and water to pan juices to make a gravy.

Top with slices of leftover chicken or other meat.

Serve over brown rice.

## MAKING IT EASY

Cooking a squash, several sweet potatoes, and a handful of beets in one session is a convenient way to ensure that these foods are ready to go and available for a few days to be assembled into a lunch bowl or plate. Whether you use starchy vegetables or not, make sure to serve a generous portion of nonstarchy vegetable alongside. You may like to precook a protein such as chicken or steak (or, if you are vegetarian, beans or legumes) and keep that ready for easy lunches too. In all cases, follow the three-day rule: Use the cooked food from the refrigerator within three days. Cook, store, take out a few hours before using to allow food to reach room temperature, then reheat before eating with a quick steam or, if you are at work or pressed for time, a quick reheat in a microwave, as long as you are not using plastic. Glass is always preferred when using a microwave. (Although microwaves are controversial, Dr. Parcells used a microwave. She said the food is cooked from the inside out, and often when there is weak digestion in the case of the elderly, the food becomes more digestible.)

# One-Bowl Salad

This is one of the tastiest ways to put together a salad meal for one person—or more if you are feeding a group. Use whatever kinds of greens, vegetables, and herbs you like!

**Extra-virgin olive oil**

**Apple cider vinegar or lemon juice**

**Sea salt**

**Fresh black pepper**

**Fresh herbs (such as parsley, chives, scallions, dill, basil, mint, or marjoram)**

**1–2 cloves garlic, mashed (optional)**

**Onions (optional)**

**Salad greens**

**Mixed vegetables of your choice, cooked or raw**

**Protein of your choice (optional)**

I always eyeball the amounts here, depending on the size of the salad bowl used. Pour a small pool of oil into the bottom of a wooden salad bowl, then pour a generous splash of apple cider vinegar or lemon juice into the oil. It will look like a sunnyside up egg, with the vinegar as the yolk in the middle that does not blend until whisked. (If you prefer measurements, for a sizable salad bowl, mix $1/4$–$1/2$ cup olive oil to $1/8$–$1/4$ cup vinegar or lemon.) Season with salt and pepper and start to stir with a wire whisk. Add fresh herbs to marinate in dressing. Tear salad greens and place these and other vegetables (if using) on top of the dressing. Right before you are ready to serve, toss the dressing up from the bottom of the bowl. You can top off with grilled chicken, poached egg, grilled salmon, or slices of leftover beef to make a meal.

# HARMONIC HEALING RECIPES

The following recipes will help you enjoy your Liver-Clear
gram and give you delicious choices for year-round cuisine.
these recipes work for the strict phase of the Liver-Cleansing Diet but,
where noted, are suitable only for the modified phase. (Remember that
vegetarians may eat grains on the strict phase.) Those on the Candida
Protocol will not use vinegars where they are called for—note the sub-
stitution listed, which is usually lemon.

## The Liver-Cleansing Drink

Used daily for the first three weeks of cleansing, this drink should be consumed
as your first food of the day and taken with no other food. Let it digest for two
hours before eating.

**1 grapefruit or orange,
peeled and chopped**
(note: use orange instead of grapefruit if
taking prescribed medications for which
grapefruit is contraindicated)

**1 lemon, peeled and chopped**

**1–2 tbsp. cold-pressed olive oil**
(start with a little less, and add more as
your taste buds acclimate and become
able to tolerate it)

**Small pinch cayenne pepper**

**1–2 garlic cloves**
(if you must avoid garlic breath due
to your work situation, use 2–4 garlic
capsules, available at health-food stores,
and swallow with your drink)

**1–2 tsp. ground flaxseed**

**$1/2$-1-inch slice fresh ginger**

Place all ingredients in a blender and add about $1/2$ cup of water—or enough to
blend into a thick drink. (Do not cover with water, or it will be too thin.) Add
more water as needed.

Blend on high until garlic, ginger, and ground flaxseed are thoroughly blended.

Drink slowly, mixing the drink with your saliva before swallowing. Drink should
be thick enough to chew. It is recommended that you make the drink fresh each
morning. It does not store well for the next day due to oxidation.

# Green Liver-Cleansing Drink

This recipe should be used as an alternative to the standard Liver-Cleansing Drink if acidity is an issue, for example if you are prone to acid reflux, GERD, gastric ulcers, or sensitivity to sour and citrus.

| | |
|---|---|
| ½ cucumber | 1 green apple |
| 2–3 celery stalks | ½ cup parsley |

Place all ingredients in a blender with enough water to blend into a thick drink. (Do not cover with water, or it will be too thin.)

Blend on high until ingredients are thoroughly blended. Drink slowly, mixing the drink with your saliva before swallowing. Drink should be thick enough to chew. It is recommended that you make the drink fresh each morning. It does not store well for the next day due to oxidation. You may follow this drink with a breakfast if desired from the allowed foods on the Strict Liver-Cleansing Diet list if you desire.

# Liver-Cleansing Tea

Use this tea as a warming "chaser" to the Liver-Cleansing Drink and, if you choose, continue to sip throughout the day, warm or at room temperature.

| | |
|---|---|
| 4–5 slices ginger | 1 tsp. fennel |
| 1 tsp. fenugreek | 1 tsp. flax seeds |
| 1 tsp. peppermint leaf | 1 inch piece of licorice root (optional) |

Boil gingerroot in 1 quart of water for 10–15 minutes. Add remaining ingredients. Turn off heat and cover. Steep for 10–15 minutes, filter through a tea strainer, then drink.

# BREAKFAST DISHES

Here are three of my favorite egg breakfasts that can be used during the Liver-Cleansing Program.

## Vegetable Frittata

The great thing about a fritatta or baking eggs is that you can use whatever left-over cooked veggies you have in the refrigerator as the star ingredient of your breakfast. If you have leftover Ratatouille (page 237), grilled vegetables, or even stir-fried Asian vegetables, they can be added to your baked egg mixture so they don't go to waste. Or you can always cook up a mixture of uncooked vegetables that you have available. The following recipe is one of my favorite combinations.

| | |
|---|---|
| 8 eggs | 6 Swiss chard leaves, chopped |
| 1 tbsp. grapeseed oil | 12 cherry tomatoes, halved |
| 2 garlic cloves, minced | Salt and pepper |
| 10 shiitake mushrooms, sliced | |

Preheat the oven to 350°F. Whisk eggs in a bowl with $1/4$ cup water. In a seasoned cast-iron skillet on stovetop at medium heat, warm grapeseed oil. Add garlic and mushrooms and cook for 3–5 minutes until mushrooms are tender. Add Swiss chard and tomatoes. Cook until wilted. Add salt and pepper to taste. Add whisked eggs to cooked vegetable mixture. Place in oven and cook for 20–30 minutes. Poke center of frittata to check if cooked through and not wet to determine when ready. Remove from oven, let sit for 5–10 minutes, then remove from skillet. Slice like a pie and serve.

## Garden Huevos Rancheros

2 tsp. ghee (divided)

2 cups cooked black beans
(for instructions, see Cuban Black
Bean Soup, page 228)

4 cups Calabacitas with
Fresh Green Chilies (page 239)

4 eggs

4 corn tortillas (omit during Strict
Liver-Cleansing Diet)

1 head romaine lettuce, shredded

$1/2$ cucumber, diced

2 tomatoes, diced

1 cup Salsa Fresca/Pico de Gallo
(page 260)

2 cups Traditional Guacamole
(page 262)

$1/2$ cup cilantro, chopped

Sea salt and fresh black pepper

I often make this as a breakfast or lunch to utilize leftovers from Southwestern-inspired dinners. If you have black beans, calabacitas, salsa, and guacamole already made, this is a perfect way to repurpose those ingredients into a delicious breakfast.

Heat 1 teaspoon ghee in a saucepan on medium heat, then add black beans. Once warm, mash beans to create a "refried" texture.

Warm calabacitas in a cast-iron skillet.

The eggs can be cooked "al gusto" (as you like), but I prefer sunny-side up. Take 1 tsp ghee and warm in a cast-iron skillet or sauté pan at medium-low heat. Break the eggs into the pan. Cook without flipping until the whites are completely cooked through and the yolks are still runny. When done, remove from heat and let sit on a plate. Warm corn tortillas in the pan, if using.

Now the fun part, building the plate layer by layer: optional corn tortilla on the bottom, then $1/2$ cup beans, 1 cup calabacitas, shredded lettuce, cucumber, tomatoes, 1 egg; top with salsa, guacamole, and cilantro. Sprinkle with sea salt and fresh black pepper to taste.

# Egg in a Kale Nest with Sweet Potato Hash

1 tbsp. grapeseed oil

$1/2$ sweet onion, diced

1 red bell pepper, diced

1 sweet potato, peeled and diced

6 kale leaves, chopped

2 cloves garlic, minced

pinch of red chili flakes

Salt and pepper

2 eggs

In a cast-iron skillet, heat grapeseed oil on medium heat. Add onion, bell pepper, and sweet potato. Cook for about 20 minutes until done. (Tip: If you have leftover cooked sweet potato, this process is much quicker.) Add salt and pepper to taste. Remove sweet potato hash from the pan and keep warm in a bowl. Add kale, garlic, and red chili flakes to the pan. Cook for about 3 minutes until starting to wilt. Form two kale "nests" using your spatula and wooden spoon. Break an egg into each nest. Cook for 3 minutes, then flip each nest to cook the top side through to desired doneness. Salt and pepper to taste. Combine with sweet potato hash on your plate.

# SAVORY BLENDED DRINKS

Use the following blended drinks to tide you over between meals or enjoy similarly to a soup as part of a vegetable-forward meal during the Liver-Cleansing Program and anytime you seek to rest and nourish the body with minimal digestive effort. They are fast to prepare and require minimal cook time. If you are doing your cleanse in the summertime, you may find that blended soups and drinks from the garden, like gazpacho, make regular appearances in your program, giving concentrated vital nutrition. You can make them with a loose hand—exact amounts are not important. Use as snacks or as a very light meal.

## Blended Salad

This can be taken before meals or on its own as a midmorning or midafternoon snack.

½ cucumber

½ tomato

Juice of half a lemon

1 tbsp. extra-virgin olive oil

4–6 dark green romaine lettuce leaves

3 celery stalks

In blender, place cucumber, tomato (if in season), lemon juice, and olive oil. Begin blending, then, while blender is running, add romaine lettuce and celery stalks. (Take off central cap of blender lid, push lettuce down using celery stalks, then replace cap.) Blend until smooth and drink immediately. You can modify this drink according to what you have on hand—avocado, parsley, cilantro, green or red peppers, scallions, and jalapeño, if desired.

## Garden Tomato Drink

4–6 medium tomatoes

1/4 cup parsley

1 tbsp. extra-virgin olive oil

1 tbsp. dulse flakes

Salt and pepper

Use the ripest tomatoes you can find (garden-grown are preferred). Place tomatoes, parsley, olive oil, and dulse flakes in the blender. Blend until liquid. You can use any of your favorite vegetable seasonings instead of dulse flakes. Add salt and pepper to taste. Drink immediately.

## Vital Broth

1 tsp. organic vegetable broth powder (e.g., Better than Bouillon or Frontier Herb)

1 1/2 cups hot water

1 cup parsley

1 cup watercress

1 cup leafy greens (e.g., Swiss chard, spinach)

In a blender, combine organic vegetable broth powder with hot water. Add parsley, watercress, and leafy greens. Blend until smooth, adding more water if needed to liquefy. Drink immediately.

# Quick Zucchini Soup

I discovered this soup as a young mother preparing "first foods" for my baby son. I would eat spoonfuls in between feeding him his, which is how I realized my baby food was a delicious gourmet soup. I frequently serve it to friends and family at my kitchen counter in the summer when zucchini are abundant, because of the healing, gelatinous nature of zucchini.

**6 small zucchini, cut into 1-inch rounds**

**1 tbsp. extra-virgin olive oil, plus more for drizzling**

**Salt and pepper**

Place zucchini in a heavy-bottomed pan (such as a Dutch oven) and add about 2 inches of water. Cover and cook on low until zucchini are translucent, about 10 minutes.

Be careful not to put too much water in the pan. It does not need to cover the zucchini. The small amount of water will retain the sweet flavor of the zucchini (and any other squash you cook this way). Place cooked zucchini into blender with olive oil. You can add some of the cooking water if needed. Pulse blender until zucchini are roughly broken up, not a completely smooth liquid. This gives the soup texture. Serve immediately. Finish with a drizzle of extra-virgin olive oil added at the table with a few flakes of sea salt and fresh ground pepper to taste. This makes a delicious starter before any meal on any program.

## Raw-Beet Borscht

1 cup beets, washed and diced

³/₄ cup raw carrots, diced

¹/₄ cup raw cucumber, diced

1 small onion, sliced

1 cup Vegetable Broth (page 220)

1 tbsp. lemon juice

Dash of sea salt

1 tsp. vegetable seasoning such as Herbamare

Blend all ingredients until smooth, adding more water or vegetable broth if needed. Taste and add more seasoning if desired. Serve warm or cold and garnish with sliced cucumber and dill or a spoonful of yogurt or sour cream (during the maintenance phase).

## Gazpacho Soup

This cold and refreshing summertime soup is a favorite at my home.

3 lbs. tomatoes, cored and coarsely chopped

1 seedless cucumber, peeled and coarsely chopped

2 red bell peppers, coarsely chopped

1 jalapeño, seeded and coarsely chopped

¹/₂ cup flat-leaf parsley

¹/₄ cup apple cider vinegar (or lemon juice)

¹/₂ cup extra-virgin olive oil

1 small sweet onion, chopped

2 cloves garlic

Sea salt and ground black pepper

In a blender, combine all ingredients, puree the vegetables until smooth, season with salt and pepper and serve.

# SLOW-SIMMERED SOUPS

During a period of cleansing and rebuilding, it is good to start a meal with soup or hot broth for concentrated nutrition. Its warmth stimulates the stomach, stimulates the digestive juices, and provides liquid to further help the digestive force. Soups can also be your meal on their own, especially substantial ones such as Grandma's Chicken Soup (page 222) or Yogi Bhajan's Mung Beans and Rice (page 233).

## Broths

Broths are wonderful healing foods to have on hand in the refrigerator or freezer. Reheat and sip for warming nourishment, or turn them into the world's easiest vegetable soups in one more simple step. The following three recipes can be done by eyeballing ingredients—you do not need exact measurements for them to work out fine. The idea is to use what you have on hand, relax, and enjoy results that are perfectly imperfect. Bon appetit!

### VEGETABLE BROTH

Fill your largest stainless-steel stock pot ¾ full of water and boil on high heat. Add a generous variety of vegetables—whatever you have on hand. Onions, celery, carrots, zucchini, potatoes, winter squashes, green beans, lettuce or green leafy vegetables, parsnips, turnips, and celery root are all good. You want enough vegetables to fill at least a third of the pot. Herbs like parsley and dill may also be added. Let simmer, partially covered, for at least 1 hour. Let cool, then strain through a fine colander into glass jars. This broth will last five days in your refrigerator or can freeze in containers for up to three months.

### BONE BROTH

Fill one third of the bottom of your largest stainless-steel pot or a large crock pot with bones and knuckles of beef or lamb. Add the trinity: 1 onion, 3 carrots, and 3 stalks celery and enough water to cover the bones and fill the pot to two inches below the brim. Cover and simmer for 24–36 hours, strain and refrigerate broth for making other soups for added calcium, magnesium, manganese, chlorine, and fluorine. Bone broth is known to be anti-inflammatory. This broth will last in glass jars for 3–4 days in your refrigerator or can freeze in containers for up to 3 months.

## ONE-STEP VEGETABLE SOUP

Use your vegetable or bone stock to make a quick vegetable soup. Add fresh diced vegetables to a pan of heated broth and allow to simmer. I typically add the holy trinity and whatever other vegetables look good that day. It can be one vegetable on its own, such as broccoli cooked until tender, or a medley. Bok choy, zucchini, spinach, Swiss chard, leeks, and watercress are good choices. Simmer until vegetables are soft but not mushy, about 30 minutes, add sea salt and pepper as desired, sprinkle with parsley or chives, and serve.

### TIP:

Hot broth may be enhanced with a spoonful of miso paste, well stirred in, and a sprinkle of seaweed such as dulse flakes for a delicious drink that is nutritious and, also important, helps to neutralize radiation. This can be especially warming as a morning drink or to wind down in the evening.

# Grandma's Chicken Soup

You barely need a recipe to make chicken soup. Just gather the ingredients and put them in a big pot . . . and let the fire do the rest. This soup is a nourishing meal anytime and is indispensable during illness or recovery from illness. Organic chicken is best, or use the Clorox Food Bath before using a non-organic chicken. This makes a healthy weekly meal for the whole family.

1 whole chicken

1 onion, peeled

3 stalks celery

3 carrots

1 bunch parsley or dill

2 tsp. sea salt

Fresh ground black pepper, at least 5 twists on the grinder

Generous splash of apple cider vinegar

1 bunch escarole or spinach

Place chicken in a large pot. Add onion, celery, carrots, parsley and/or dill. Cover with at least 3-4 inches of water over the top of the chicken and veggies, add sea salt and black pepper, apple cider vinegar, and let simmer for 2–3 hours.

Remove chicken from pot and set aside to cool. Meanwhile, strain broth.

When chicken is cool enough to touch, pull it apart, taking all the meat off the bones (being careful to remove all tiny bones and gristle). Set meat aside.

Bring broth to a simmer and add handfuls of torn escarole or spinach. Simmer until the greens are tender, then add chicken back to soup. Optional: well-cooked brown rice can be added when serving. If you are on the strict phase, omit but make the brown rice for the family to enjoy in their soup.

# Dr. Linda's Italian Lentil Soup

Another go-to in my house is lentil soup. Economical, tasty, and hearty, this lentil soup fills the stomach and the soul for both vegetarians and meat eaters!

$1^1/_2$ cups green lentils, or Umbrian or French lentils

2 large carrots, diced or in chunks

2 stalks celery, cut into half-inch slices

1 whole onion, diced

3 fresh tomatoes or 1 16-oz jar whole organic tomatoes

1 tsp. dried basil

$^1/_2$ tsp. dried oregano

$^1/_2$ tsp. dried marjoram

Splash apple cider vinegar (or lemon juice)

Good-size pinch sea salt

4–5 turns of the black pepper grinder

A few cloves smashed garlic

Wash the lentils thoroughly in water, then drain. Place all ingredients in a heavy pot. Cover about 5 inches over the top of lentils and cook at low heat for at least one hour. Taste and check if lentils are tender, adding more water as needed, depending how thick or thin you like your soup. When lentils are tender, you can add greens like escarole or spinach and let cook another 15 minutes. (I like to keep my lentil soup thin and add a whole head of escarole toward the end of cooking.) When serving, drizzle extra-virgin olive oil on top and sprinkle with sea salt, give a splash of apple cider vinegar and freshly ground pepper. Optional: top with freshly-grated Parmesan cheese, if desired.

TIP:

A salad of Boston lettuce with a simple lemon and olive oil dressing or Harmonic Beet Salad (page 234) can be served with the Italian lentil soup to make a nice meal.

# Red Lentil Soup

Another staple soup, this one can be modified with any kind of vegetables you have on hand. If you are eating grains, it can be served with plain basmati or brown or red rice, and it goes well with a vegetable dish such as Indian-Style Cabbage Bhaji (page 235) or any steamed vegetables.

$1\frac{1}{2}$ cups red lentils (picked over for debris or stones)

1 onion, cut into chunks

$\frac{1}{2}$ tsp. ground cumin

1–2 tbsp. finely chopped ginger

1 small green chili, diced, seeds removed (optional)

1–2 cups any vegetables (green beans, broccoli, carrots, celery, zucchini, peas, etc.)

1 tsp. sea salt

1 tbsp. grapeseed oil or ghee

1 tsp. black mustard seeds

$\frac{1}{2}$ tsp. fenugreek seeds

3 cloves garlic, chopped

$\frac{1}{2}$ cup slivered onions

1 lemon wedge

Wash the lentils thoroughly in water, then drain. Fill a pot with about 9 cups water and bring to a boil. Add lentils, then bring back to boil stirring, then turn heat down to simmer. Cook about half an hour without cover. Stir in onion chunks, cumin, ginger, chili (if using), and vegetables. Cover and cook until lentils are soft, about another half hour or so. Add salt. In a heavy frying pan, heat grapeseed oil or ghee and drop in one mustard seed. If it pops, add the remaining mustard seeds and then the fenugreek seeds, stirring constantly. Turn heat down and add garlic and slivered onions. Add to lentils and simmer to blend tastes. Optional: Add a squeeze of lemon juice.

# French Peasant Soup with Pistou

This is an adaptation of a recipe I discovered while watching Julia Child on television as a child. I was always fascinated by French cooking, so I began studying her methods. I have made this soup for decades, and I get rave reviews from family and friends every time I make it! *Pistou* is French for a savory paste known in Italy as "pesto." This soup is delightful as a meal served in a large bowl (with sourdough bread during the maintenance phase) alongside a green salad. Or serve as a starter before an entrée of protein, such as a grilled chicken breast or beef fillet, with a salad.

3 quarts water

2 tbsp. sea salt

2 cups diced carrots

2 cups diced potatoes

2 cups diced sweet onions or leeks

2 cups green beans

1–2 cups fresh zucchini, peas, and or red or green peppers

1 cup cooked cannellini or kidney beans (optional)

4 tbsp. fresh flat-leaf parsley, chopped

## PISTOU FLAVORING:

4 cloves garlic

4 tbsp. tomato paste

1/4 cup fresh basil

1/2 cup grated Parmesan cheese (optional, for use during maintenance phase only)

1/2 cup extra-virgin olive oil

In a four-quart pot, simmer water, salt, carrots, potatoes, and onions or leeks uncovered for 40 minutes. Add green beans, zucchini, peas, and/or red or green peppers, and cannellini or kidney beans (if using) to the slow-boiling base. Cook for another 15 minutes or until green beans are tender. Meanwhile, prepare the pistou flavoring in a soup tureen or other pot. Press garlic, then stir in tomato paste, basil, and optional Parmesan. Then with a wire whisk, gradually beat in olive oil by droplets to make a thick paste. Dribble several ladlefuls of hot soup into pistou and gradually stir in rest of soup. Stir in parsley and serve.

# Passato di Verdure (Churned Vegetable Soup)

This is one of my favorite soups! My dear friend and New York restaurateur Beatrice Tosti, has perfected the recipe, and we have made it our "go-to soup" for high-concentrated nutrition. *Passato* comes from *passaverdure*, which means "hand-churned" in Italian. You may use any green vegetable you want but can also add tomatoes and/or root vegetables. The vegetables can change with the season and can be served hot or cold. Extra-virgin olive oil can be drizzled on the soup after cooking for added flavor and nutrition. You may also add cooked rice (if using grains) or a poached egg on top when serving.

½ cup extra-virgin olive oil

1 bunch Swiss chard, carefully washed and shredded by hand

1 bunch spinach, carefully washed and shredded by hand

1 bunch dandelion greens, carefully washed and shredded by hand

1 bunch Tuscan kale (or Russian kale, depending on season), stems removed, carefully washed and shredded by hand

2 carrots, coarsely chopped

1 onion, coarsely chopped

5 shallots, coarsely chopped

5 cloves garlic

1 heart of celery, white part only, coarsely chopped

1 tbsp. sea salt (or more to taste)

Crushed red chili flakes to taste

Place your heaviest and largest stock pot on your stove. Add oil, all greens, and all chopped vegetables. Add sea salt and the crushed chili flakes and barely cover with water (you can always add more water later). Bring to a slow boil, then lower the heat to a low simmer, place a lid over pot, and let cook for 1–1½ hours. (Do not sauté the vegetables and the greens first. It all goes into the pot at the same time. In Italy this soup is cooked slowly all day on the side of the fire.) Taste for seasoning, remove from heat, and turn into a *passato* or blended soup, using an immersion blender if possible, and otherwise hand-churning with a fork.

# Cannellini Bean and Escarole Soup

Coming from an Italian household, I grew to love all kinds of beans served with bitter greens. My favorite is the white bean. Here is a recipe I use as a complete meal or as a side dish.

1½ cups cannellini, or great northern, gigante, or other white beans

2 quarts water

2 bay leaves

½ cup extra-virgin olive oil (divided)

Sea salt

6 cups escarole leaves (preferably tough outer leaves), coarsely shredded, washed, and drained

8 garlic cloves, peeled and cut in half

6 whole dried pepperoncini (hot red peppers)

The night before: It's always a good idea to pick over dried beans to remove any dirt or tiny stones. Then dump the beans into a 2- to 3-quart container and pour in enough cold water to cover them by at least four inches. Let soak in a cool place at least 8 hours or up to 24 hours. Drain thoroughly. When time is limited, a jar of cooked cannellini beans can be used instead.

Drain and transfer beans to a 5- or 6-quart pot. Pour in the 2 quarts of water, toss in bay leaves, and bring to a boil. Adjust heat to a simmer, pour in ¼ cup of the olive oil, and cook until beans are tender, 1–1½ hours. By the time the beans are tender, they should be covered by about one inch of cooking liquid. Season beans to taste with salt. Stir in escarole and cook, stirring occasionally, until escarole is quite tender, about 20–30 minutes. Remove the pot from the heat.

Heat the remaining ¼ cup oil in a small skillet over very low heat, add the garlic and pepperoncini, and cook, shaking the pan, until the pepperoncini change color, about 1 minute or less. Remove from heat and carefully pour one ladleful of soup into the skillet (it will sputter quite a bit). Swirl the pan to blend the two, then stir the panful of seasoned soup back into the large pot. Check the seasoning and let the soup rest off the heat, covered, 10–15 minutes. Serve with garlic bread if you like (during the maintenance phase).

# Cuban Black Bean Soup

Black bean soup is satisfying on its own, as a main course with a grain, or modified by adding avocado, sliced red onion, a poached egg, or some goat cheese on top. You can also use leftovers to make refried black beans. This recipe is broken into two steps—basic black beans to use in other dishes and black bean soup made with sofrito, an aromatic sauce that is common in Caribbean cuisine.

1 lb. dried black beans, rinsed, picked over for stones, and soaked overnight

$1\frac{1}{2}$ green peppers, stemmed and seeded

4 garlic cloves

2 bay leaves

1 tbsp. sea salt

$\frac{1}{4}$ cup extra-virgin olive oil

1 onion, diced

1 jalapeño, stemmed and finely chopped

1 tsp. dried oregano or 1 tbsp. fresh oregano

$\frac{1}{2}$ tsp. ground cumin

$\frac{1}{2}$ tsp. freshly ground black pepper

3 tbsp. apple cider vinegar (or lemon or lime juice)

$\frac{1}{2}$ green pepper, stemmed and seeded

6 garlic cloves

2 tsp. sea salt plus additional as needed to taste

**STEP 1:** Make the basic black beans. Cut 1 of the green peppers into 1-inch squares. Smash and peel 4 of the garlic cloves. Put the green pepper and garlic into a large pot with the black beans, 2 bay leaves, and 1 tablespoon salt. Add 2 quarts water and bring to a boil. Cover the pot and simmer until the beans are tender, at least an hour or more.

**STEP 2:** Make the sofrito. Cut the remaining half of green pepper into quarter-inch pieces. Peel and chop the rest of the garlic. Heat the olive oil in a large skillet over low heat (grapeseed oil is a fine alternative). Cook, stirring occasionally, until it starts to brown, about 5 minutes. Add the green pepper and onion and cook, stirring, until softened, about 5 minutes. Add the garlic, jalapeño (leave out the seeds if you don't want your soup too spicy), oregano, cumin, black pepper, and 2 teaspoons salt and stir for a few minutes. Pour in the vinegar and scrape any browned bits from bottom of the pan with a wooden spoon. This is your sofrito.

When the beans are cooked, discard the bay leaf. Transfer 1 cup of beans to a small bowl, mash into a paste with the back of a fork, and return to the pot. Add the sofrito.

Stir in the rest of the beans and bring to a slow boil, then lower to a simmer and let cook, uncovered, for another 20 minutes or so, skimming any foam that may have gathered from the top. Taste for salt and serve over basmati or well-cooked brown rice and guacamole.

# Dr. Linda's Dal with Veggies

This is my basic dal recipe, which I have used for the last forty-plus years. It can be modified according to the season and what looks good in the market. It can be a staple of your Liver-Cleansing Program whether you are a vegetarian or an omnivore. Lentils come in many varieties, yellow, white, or red. Red is traditional and works very well in this recipe.

1 cup lentils, picked over for stones

1 tbsp. ghee

1/4 tsp. black mustard seeds

1/4 tsp. coriander seeds

1/4 tsp. fenugreek seeds

1/2 tsp. ground cumin

1 tsp. turmeric

2 cloves garlic, chopped

1 knob fresh ginger, chopped

1 large onion, chopped

1/4 -1/2 tsp. ground cayenne powder according to taste

1 tsp. sea salt and more to taste

4 curry leaves

2/3 cup carrots, chopped

2 small zucchini, cut into small chunks

10 green beans, cut into 1-inch pieces

Any greens available in your refrigerator according to season, chopped

Wash the lentils thoroughly in water, then drain. Heat ghee over medium heat. Add black mustard seeds, coriander, and fenugreek. When mustard seeds begin to pop, add cumin, turmeric, garlic, ginger, and onion. Let this blend cook until onions are translucent. Add cayenne and salt. Then add curry leaves, lentils, carrots, zucchini, and string beans. Add water to cover and cook for about 1 hour, adding enough water to make a loose/thin dal. Add greens (kale, Swiss chard, spinach, broccoli, or any other green vegetable you like) and continue to cook until tender. Taste for seasoning and add more sea salt if needed.

# Dr. Linda's Kitchari

Kitchari is a very cleansing food in Ayurveda. Incredibly simple to digest, it allows the whole digestive system to rest and restore. The gift of kitchari is that the vegetables can be varied according to season. It is a staple food in the vegetarian diet because the balance of the grain and legume makes a complete protein. If you are on the first three weeks of the Liver-Cleansing Diet (the strict phase), you would normally not be eating grains, but kitchari can be used as the protein portion of your meal during both phases of the Liver-Cleansing Diet because of its ease of digestion.

1 cup split mung beans (see note below)

1 cup basmati rice

1 yellow onion, chopped

1 square inch fresh ginger, chopped

3 cloves garlic, chopped

2 stalks celery, chopped

3 carrots, chopped

2 stalks broccoli, chopped (or chopped kale, spinach, zucchini, green beans, or any vegetable in season)

1 heaping tsp. turmeric

$1/4$ tsp. cayenne

1 tsp. Basic Curry Powder, if desired (recipe page 232)

1 tsp. cumin seeds or ajwan seeds

Fill a pot with 3 quarts of water and bring to a boil. Keep a slow boil going, add all ingredients, partially cover, and cook for 20 minutes or more. The pot can overflow easily and you may need to add more water, depending on if you want your kitchari soupy or thick. Stir from time to time. When all ingredients are merged, let kitchari sit to cool for 20 minutes. It will thicken up on its own. Serve with freshly ground pepper and sea salt, and top with some ghee or olive oil, chopped cilantro, or parsley.

**NOTE:** If you use whole mung beans instead of split ones, they must be boiled until quite mushy, 30–45 minutes, before adding other ingredients.

## Basic Curry Powder

1 tsp. ground turmeric

1 tsp. cumin seeds

1 tsp. coriander seeds

4 or more whole cloves

2 cardamom pods

1 tsp. or more chili powder or ground dried chili pepper

Grind all ingredients together in a mortar and pestle, and mix to combine.

# Yogi Bhajan's Mung Beans and Rice

"Bold and hearty, rich and nourishing. Just like Yogi Ji" is how I describe this soup, which Yogi Bhajan required all students to eat during Kundalini yoga teacher training. In fact, he often put his students on mung beans and rice for forty days at a time, with no other foods allowed, due to its cleansing nature. If you are vegetarian, turn to this recipe often during your entire Liver-Cleansing Program, as it is easy to digest. If you are not, it is ideal during the modified phase.

1 cup whole mung beans (presoaked 4–6 hours)

1 cup basmati rice

4–6 cups chopped assorted vegetables (carrots, celery, zucchini, broccoli, green beans, etc.), in small pieces

1 tbsp. ghee

2 small onions, chopped

8 cloves garlic

1/3 cup minced fresh ginger

1 tsp. turmeric

1/2 tsp. fresh ground black pepper

1 heaping tsp. garam masala

1 tsp. crushed red chili flakes

2 bay leaves

Seeds of 5 cardamom pods

1 tsp. dried sweet basil

Sea salt to taste

1/4 cup fresh cilantro, chopped, for garnish

Rinse beans and rice separately until water runs clear, then set aside. Bring about 9 cups of water to a boil, add rice and beans, and let boil over medium flame. Add vegetables to the cooking rice and beans. Heat ghee in a skillet. Add the onions, garlic, and ginger and sauté over low heat until starts to turn brown. Add the spices except the basil and sea salt and cook for a minute or two. Add this mixture and the basil to the rice-and-beans. Stir often to prevent scorching, and add water if needed. Continue to cook over low heat for at least 1 hour until beans are tender and the consistency is rich, thick, and soup-like. Add sea salt to taste and serve garnished with chopped cilantro.

# COOKED VEGETABLE DISHES

## Harmonic Beet Salad

Friends and family always ask me to bring my famous beet salad to potluck dinners. The simple combination of tender, sweet, juicy beets with sour apple cider vinegar and pungent red onion excites the taste buds and promotes digestion.

4 beets, cooked, steamed, peeled, and sliced (Simple Steamed Beets, page 203)

$^1/_2$ medium red onion, diced, or 2–3 garlic cloves, minced

1 tbsp. fresh flat-leaf parsley or dill, minced

1–2 tbsp. apple cider vinegar (or lemon juice)

$^1/_2$ tsp. honey (optional)

2–3 tbsp. extra-virgin olive oil

Sea salt to taste

Place beets and onion or garlic in a bowl. While tossing, add parsley or dill, apple cider vinegar, honey (if using), and enough olive oil to form dressing. Add sea salt to taste. Chill and serve later.

# Indian-Style Cabbage Bhaji

If cabbage is not your favorite vegetable, get creative here: Any vegetable can be cooked in this classic Indian vegetable dish. Cauliflower is a great one to try. Served with a grain and a bean or with meat, chicken, or fish, it makes a wonderful meal.

2 cups chopped cabbage

1 tbsp. ghee

$1/2$ tsp. cumin seeds

12 curry leaves

1 green chili, chopped

1 pinch asafoetida (hing) powder (specialty spice found at Asian grocers; helps with gas)

Sea salt to taste

2 tbsp. chopped fresh cilantro

Rinse and slice or shred cabbage.

Heat ghee in a shallow frying pan. Add cumin seeds and let them sputter or dance around the pan exploding flavor. Then add curry leaves, chopped green chili, and asafoetida. Stir to mix well. Add cabbage to pan with a cup of water and cover. Stir periodically, if you see the cabbage getting brown, add a little more water. Cook on low heat until cabbage is tender. Turn off flame, add sea salt to taste and fresh cilantro, mix well, and serve.

# Bright Yellow Cashew Rice

When grains are added back into your diet on the Modified phase of the liver cleanse, try this vibrant and anti-inflammatory turmeric-spiked dish. Vegetarians may enjoy it throughout the six weeks. For a complete Indian-inspired meal, serve with the Dr. Linda's Dal with Veggies (page 230) and Indian-Style Cabbage Bhaji (page 235).

$1/2$ cup raw cashews

2 medium onions, diced

1 tbsp. ghee

1 cup uncooked organic brown rice (long- or short-grain)

1 tsp. ground turmeric

2 cups water

1 tsp. sea salt

4–5 scallions, chopped

Lightly toast cashews in a cast-iron pan and set aside. In a medium heavy pot, sauté onions in ghee, stir in rice, and continue cooking for a few minutes. Sprinkle in turmeric and stir quickly to avoid burning. Add water and sea salt and bring to a boil. Simmer, covered, for 45 minutes. Toss in cashews and scallions before serving.

# Ratatouille

Vegetable stews such as ratatouille are a simple way to bring new flavors to the table. This is a favorite in summer, when the garden is bursting with beautiful ingredients.

2 large onions, sliced

2 large cloves garlic, minced or mashed

1 medium eggplant, cut into half-inch cubes

6 medium zucchini, thickly sliced

2 green or red peppers, seeded and cut in chunks

2 tsp. sea salt

1 tsp. dried basil or 3 tbsp. minced fresh basil

1/2 cup minced parsley

4 large fresh tomatoes, cut in chunks

4 tbsp. extra-virgin olive oil

1/4 cup fresh parsley leaves, for garnish

1 tomato, sliced, for garnish

Layer all ingredients except olive oil and garnishes in a 6-quart Dutch oven, pressing down to make fit. Drizzle olive oil over top layer, cover casserole, and bake at 325°F for 3 hours.

Uncover during last hour, mix gently, and salt to taste. Serve hot or cold. Garnish with parsley and sliced tomato.

# Mixed Vegetable Curry

You get the healing benefits of many different spices in this dish—and it's as easy as one, two, three to prepare.

1 cup cauliflower, cut into medium-sized pieces

1 cup diced carrots

2 cups green beans, cut into 1-inch pieces

1 cup green peas, fresh or frozen (see note below)

2 tbsp. ghee

2 tsp. cumin seeds

1 tsp. sea salt

2 tsp. mustard seeds

2 tsp. turmeric

1 tsp. coriander seeds

1/2 tsp. cayenne

Slowly cook cauliflower, carrots, green beans, and peas, if using fresh, in about 2–3 inches of water. Set aside in the pot; do not drain. In a separate pot, heat ghee and stir in the spices. Add the mixed vegetables to the pot with the ghee and spices. Bring to a boil. Stir well and simmer for 20 minutes.

**NOTE:** Ordinarily I do not recommend frozen food; the occasional package of frozen peas for vegetable curry is the exception. If using frozen peas, add during the last 5 minutes of cooking.

# Calabacitas with Fresh Green Chilies

In New Mexico we are blessed to have green chilies, corn, and zucchini in abundance in the summer. This local dish is available at most New Mexican restaurants. It pairs well with eggs and works as a side dish with a protein or as the filling for an enchilada.

$1^1/_2$ lbs. zucchini (about 5 medium zucchinis)

2 tbsp. ghee

$1/_2$ cup onion, chopped

1 tbsp. minced garlic

$3/_4$ tsp. dried oregano

$1/_2$–1 cup fresh chopped green chilies

1 cup corn kernels (1 large or 2 medium ears of corn)

$1/_4$ tsp. sea salt

Freshly ground black pepper

2 tbsp. chopped cilantro

Trim the ends of the zucchini and quarter lengthwise. Cut each quarter crosswise into half-inch pieces. Set aside. Melt the ghee in a large heavy-bottomed skillet over low heat. Add the onion and cook until it softens, about 3 minutes. Stir in the garlic and the oregano and cook until fragrant, about 1 minute. Stir in zucchini and green chilies, cover tightly, and cook until the zucchini softens, about 5 minutes. Add the corn kernels and heat through, about 2 minutes. Season with about $1/_4$ teaspoon salt and a pinch of black pepper, or to taste, then remove from heat and stir in cilantro. Serve hot.

# MEDITERRANEAN QUARTET

I have always considered the Liver-Cleansing Diet to be based on the healthy Mediterranean diet. My cooking is often inspired by the flavors and ingredients of Italy, Spain, France, Morocco, Greece, and the Middle East. The daily diets of inhabitants in those regions are balanced with fresh fish, poultry, and/or lamb, fresh organic produce, herbs, spices, and olive oil. The following four recipes are side-dish staples served family style for a lunch—or a summer party. They're even better served with Homemade Hummus (page 261), Greek Salad (page 245), grilled fish, and cooked bitter greens.

## Quinoa Tabbouleh

1¹/₂ cups water

1 cup quinoa

1 cup chopped green onion or scallion

1 cup chopped fresh Italian parsley

Large pinch dried oregano

2 cloves garlic, mashed

4 stalks celery, finely chopped

1 green bell pepper, chopped

2 medium cucumbers, chopped

1 tsp. sea salt

6 tbsp. extra-virgin olive oil

8 tbsp. lemon juice

2 large tomatoes, chopped

Bring water to a boil. Rinse quinoa, then slowly add to boiling water and simmer until all water has evaporated, about 15 minutes. Set aside to cool for 2 hours. Add rest of ingredients except tomatoes, and allow to fully chill until ready to serve. Add tomatoes just before serving, because they will make the tabbouleh soggy if it sits for too long.

## Grilled Baba Ghanoush

2 medium-large eggplants (Italian or Sicilian graffiti type eggplants)

Grapeseed oil

3–4 cloves garlic, mashed

1 tsp. sea salt

2 tbsp. tahini

Juice of 1 lemon

$1/4$ cup extra-virgin olive oil

$1/2$ cup finely-minced fresh flat leaf Italian parsley

Sprinkle of sweet paprika

Preheat grill or grill pan to medium heat. Cut eggplants into $1/4$ inch spears lengthwise and drizzle with grapeseed oil. Cook on each side until tender. When cool, scrape insides out and add to a food processor or mash by hand with garlic, sea salt, tahini, lemon, and olive oil until smooth. Add parsley and sweet paprika, additional salt if needed, and olive oil and lemon to taste.

## Socca Flatbread

This gluten-free flatbread made with chickpea flour has the feeling of bread without the grains. It is tasty with soup or with a dip like Grilled Baba Ghanoush (see above) or Homemade Hummus (page 261).

2 cups chickpea flour

2 cups water

1–2 tsp. sea salt

$1/2$ cup extra-virgin olive oil, plus more to coat heated skillet

Stir chickpea flour into water to make a paste. Add sea salt and olive oil. Stir to eliminate any clumps, cover, and let sit for at least 1 hour. Preheat oven to 375°F and place a seasoned cast-iron skillet in the oven for 10 minutes. Remove skillet from oven and coat with oil. Pour batter into skillet about half an inch thick. Cook for 10 minutes or until golden brown. Remove from oven, let sit for 3–5 minutes, and serve. Fresh herbs like rosemary, chives, or thyme can be added to flavor the flatbread in different ways depending on your preference.

## Mediterranean Grilled Vegetables

About 2-3 tbsp. grapeseed oil

1 large sweet or Vidalia onion (see note below), cut into 3 thick rings

2 medium zucchini, cut lengthwise into quarters

2 summer squash, cut lengthwise into quarters

2 bell peppers, stems removed, quartered

1 medium-large Italian eggplant, cut lengthwise into sixths

Sea salt

Freshly ground black pepper

Extra-virgin olive oil to taste

Heat outdoor grill or grill pan to medium heat. Drizzle a small amount of grapeseed oil onto all veggies, or wipe a hot grill with grapeseed oil to prevent sticking. Season veggies with salt and pepper. Grill on each side until black grill marks are seen and each side is tender, about 4 minutes per side. Finish with olive oil and serve. I like to serve Jalapeño Sauce (page 259) with the Mediterranean Grill.

**NOTE ON CHOOSING ONIONS:** The flatter the onion, the sweeter it is. Globe-shaped are typically more pungent.

# SUBSTANTIAL SALADS

## Dr. Linda's Olive Oil and Lemon Dressing

This is my family's go-to dressing for most salads, since it is simple, healthy, and delicious. When in season, I use Meyer lemons, but any lemon or even lime can be used. I also prefer high-quality Mediterranean extra-virgin olive oil and good sea salt. When a recipe has very few ingredients, it is important for each one to be of superior quality.

2 tbsp. extra-virgin olive oil

Juice of 1 lemon

Sea salt and freshly ground black pepper to taste

Place all ingredients in a mixing bowl or small glass jar. Whisk or shake until the dressing has emulsified. The jar is handy because the dressing can be saved in this container.

# Grilled Chicken Paillard Salad

The trick to paillard is picking high-quality chicken and pounding out the breasts until they are extra thin. This tenderizes the meat and shortens cook time on the grill.

2 boneless, skinless chicken breasts

1/4 cup grapeseed oil

Sea salt and freshly ground black pepper to taste

Juice of 1 lemon

1 head of frisée, rinsed, dried, and chopped

2 cups baby arugula, rinsed and dried

1/2 cup radicchio, rinsed, dried, and chopped

2 cups vine-ripened cherry tomatoes, halved, or 2 heirloom tomatoes, sliced

1/2 cup fresh basil, torn or loosely chopped

3–4 oz. Dr. Linda's Olive Oil and Lemon Dressing (page 243)

Preheat grill or grill pan to medium heat. On a cutting board, clean the chicken breasts and cut each into 4–5 small to medium-sized pieces. (I find it easier to cook multiple medium-sized pieces than one very large piece of breast.) Place each piece in a separate ziplock or other plastic bag and pound with the flat side of a meat tenderizer, a mallet, or a rolling pin to a 1/2 inch thickness. Drizzle with grapeseed oil and season with salt and pepper. Just before placing on a hot grill or grill pan, drizzle with lemon juice. Cook for about 4 minutes on each side, until dark grill marks appear and chicken is cooked through.

In a salad bowl, combine greens, tomatoes, and basil (save a pinch of this for garnish), and mix together with the dressing.

Place cooked chicken on bottom of plate and pile salad on top. Finish with salt, pepper, and a pinch of basil on top.

## Greek Salad

1 head romaine lettuce, chopped

1 English cucumber, halved lengthwise and cut into 1 inch pieces

1 green bell pepper, deseeded and cut into 1 inch pieces

2 stalks celery, cut into half-inch pieces

1 cup cherry, grape, or heirloom tomatoes, halved or cut into 1 inch pieces

1 red onion, sliced thin into half rounds

1 small jar marinated artichoke hearts

$^1/_4$ cup kalamata olives

1 cup cooked garbanzo beans

Sea salt and fresh ground black pepper to taste

3–4 oz. Dr. Linda's Olive Oil and Lemon Dressing (page 243)

$^1/_2$ cup fresh parsley, chopped

Pinch dried oregano

$^1/_2$ cup fresh sheep feta cheese, crumbled (optional)

If on Liver-Cleansing Diet, substitute feta with 4 oz. grilled chicken or grilled salmon per person

Extra-virgin olive oil to taste

Mix all ingredients except oregano and feta (or other protein) in a salad bowl. Add feta or protein on top of salad, and finish with olive oil and oregano.

# Niçoise Salad

This salad goes great with poached, grilled, steamed, or baked salmon topped with herbes de Provence and lemon, or salmon prepared in parchment paper (see page 206) with dill, lemon, and capers.

### LEMON CAPER DRESSING

2 tbsp. extra-virgin olive oil

Juice of 1 lemon

1 tsp. capers

Pinch fresh dill

1 tsp. Dijon mustard

$^1/_2$ tsp. sea salt

$^1/_2$ tsp. freshly ground black pepper

### SALAD

2 hard-boiled eggs, cut in half lengthwise

1–2 cooked beets, peeled, chilled, cut into quarter-inch rounds

4–6 fingerling potatoes, cooked, chilled, and cut in half lengthwise (optional)

4–6 stalks asparagus, blanched and halved lengthwise (see blanching instructions on page 247)

1 tbsp. extra-virgin olive oil to drizzle

Sea salt and freshly ground black pepper to taste

$^1/_2$ lb. baby spinach, washed and dried

8–12 marinated olives (Niçoise, olive oil cured, or any Mediterranean olives)

1 tbsp. capers

To make the dressing: Mix all ingredients in blender for about 2 minutes until emulsified and smooth.

Arrange hard-boiled eggs, beets, potatoes, and asparagus on a plate. Drizzle ingredients with olive oil and season with salt and pepper. In a mixing bowl, dress spinach with dressing and add on top of the plate. Finish with olives and capers spread on top.

Bring 6–8 cups of water to a rolling boil. Season water with 1–2 tablespoons sea salt. Slide rinsed and trimmed or snapped asparagus spears into boiling water. Fill a large bowl with ice water. Once asparagus has become tender, about 3–4 minutes depending on thickness, drain in a colander and place in the ice water to stop the cooking process. Let sit for about 1–2 minutes. Drain, dry, and cool in the refrigerator.

# Southwest Salad

This salad pairs beautifully with dry-rubbed and grilled mahimahi or salmon steak (see Southwest Dry Rub, page 254).

## SOUTHWEST CILANTRO LIME DRESSING

$^1/_2$ cup fresh cilantro, destemmed and chopped

2 oz. lime juice (from 1–2 limes)

2 tbsp. extra-virgin olive oil

2 dashes ground cumin

1 tsp. sea salt

$^1/_2$ tsp. freshly ground black pepper

## SALAD

1 head of romaine, chopped

$^1/_2$ English cucumber, peeled and chopped into half-inch pieces

$^1/_2$ medium jicama, peeled and chopped into half-inch pieces

2 carrots, peeled and chopped into half-inch pieces

1 avocado, skin and pit removed, cut into half-inch pieces

1 medium tomato, diced

1 mango, skin and pit removed, cut into half-inch pieces

1 cup cooked black beans (see instructions on page 228)

$^1/_4$ cup fresh cilantro, cleaned and destemmed

Dash ground cayenne pepper or sweet paprika

To make the dressing: Combine cilantro, lime juice, olive oil, cumin, salt, and pepper together and blend for about 2 minutes until emulsified and smooth.

Toss all salad ingredients together in a large bowl. Mix in the salad dressing. Finish with more fresh cilantro and a dash of cayenne or sweet paprika, depending on your taste.

# Italian Dandelion Salad

One of nature's finest liver-cleansing foods is the bitter green dandelion. This salad goes well with a frittata or baked yam and steamed beets.

## LEMON ANCHOVY DRESSING

Juice of 1 lemon

2 tbsp. extra-virgin olive oil

1 tbsp. anchovy paste

1 tsp. Dijon mustard

1 egg yolk

4 fresh basil leaves

Pinch sea salt

$1/2$ tsp. freshly ground black pepper

## SALAD

1 bunch fresh dandelion, rinsed, dried, and roughly chopped

1 cup radicchio, rinsed, dried, and roughly chopped

Freshly ground black pepper to taste

8–12 cherry tomatoes, halved (optional)

3–4 grated peels of Italian hard sheep cheese such as Pecorino Romano or parmesan cheese (optional)

Make the dressing: Mix all ingredients in a blender until emulsified and smooth.

In a salad bowl, toss greens with dressing. Finish with freshly ground black pepper to taste and optional tomatoes and grated parmesan cheese.

## Lebanese-Style Marinated Grilled Chicken

Grilled chicken works well on the program. This is an easy recipe to make for two or more people. Grilled skewered chicken has a special feeling of fun to it.

3 cloves garlic, crushed

1/4 cup extra-virgin olive oil or grapeseed oil

Juice of 1 lemon

1 6-oz. jar organic tomato paste

1 tbsp. sweet paprika

2 tbsp. za'atar spice blend or sumac

1 tsp. sea salt

2 tsp. black pepper

4 boneless, skinless chicken breasts, cut into 4–6 large chunks to be skewered

Mix together all ingredients except chicken, then add chicken. Place in a tightly sealed glass bowl to marinate for 2 or more hours or overnight in the refrigerator. Soak wooden skewers in water for 20 minutes so that they do not burn when grilled. Skewer chicken, about 4–5 pieces per skewer. Place on hot grill or grill pan at medium heat and cook on each side, turning every 3–5 minutes so that the outside develops a nice char/caramelization and the inside is cooked through. On average, the skewers will be turned about 3–4 times, and the chicken should be cooked through after about 12–15 minutes. Serve warm with Jalapeño Sauce (page 259).

# Sunday Roasted Whole Chicken

There are many ways to prepare a roasted chicken. I love roasting a chicken for Sunday dinner and am happy to have leftovers for Monday lunch.

1 whole organic, free-range chicken, 3½–4 lbs.

1 sweet potato, peeled and cut into 1½- to 2-inch chunks

1 sweet onion, outer shell removed, cut into one-inch-thick half rounds

2–4 medium carrots, cut into one-inch rounds

12 whole brussels sprouts, trimmed and outer leaves removed

2–4 baby beets, peeled and halved

2 tbsp. grapeseed oil

1 lemon

2–3 tsp. sea salt

2 tsp. freshly ground black pepper

2 tsp. herbes de Provence

Take chicken out of refrigerator and let sit at room temperature for 30 minutes before cooking. Preheat oven to 350°F. Wash chicken under cold water and pat dry with paper towel. Place chicken in a roasting pan surrounded by sweet potato, onion, carrots, brussels sprouts, and baby beets. (Other root vegetables like turnips, parsnips, and rutabaga can all be used as variations.) Drizzle a small amount of grapeseed oil and squeeze juice of lemon over chicken and vegetables, and place the juiced lemon inside the chicken's cavity. Sprinkle all with sea salt, black pepper, and herbes de Provence. (Other herb combinations can be used, like fresh thyme or rosemary.)

Roast slowly at 350°F for 1½ hours. Basting during cooking is helpful to move around the juice that has come out of the chicken. If sticking occurs, you can add additional lemon juice or a little white wine to the pan. A meat thermometer can be helpful to see when center of chicken is cooked through at 180°F. The juices that flow out when chicken is pierced with a fork should be clear.

# Spiralized Zucchini Noodles with Buffalo or Turkey Bolognese

This recipe requires a spiralizer or the purchase of spiraled zucchini, which is readily available at many supermarkets. You can roast a spaghetti squash if you do not have access to a spiralizer or prespiralized vegetables.

2 tbsp. grapeseed oil (divided)

1 tsp. dried basil

1 tsp. dried oregano

$1/2$ tsp. red chile flakes

4–5 cloves garlic, finely diced

1 lb. 93% lean ground turkey meat (or ground organic local buffalo, bison)

2 18-oz. jars whole peeled cooked tomatoes

$1/4$ cup chopped flat-leaf parsley

$1/4$ cup chopped fresh basil

Sea salt to taste

3–4 medium zucchini, spiraled

Extra-virgin olive oil, for drizzling

Warm a large saucepan or Dutch oven on the stovetop at medium-high heat. Add grapeseed oil, dried basil, oregano, and chili flakes to pan. Cook for 3 minutes to extract flavor of herbs into the oil. Add garlic and ground meat, using a spatula to break up meat as it cooks. Cook until meat is browned, about 7–10 minutes. Add whole peeled cooked tomatoes. Lower heat and simmer for 30–40 minutes. Stir in parsley and fresh basil and remove from heat. Add sea salt to taste.

In a separate heated pan, add 1 tablespoon grapeseed oil or $1/2$ cup of water. On medium heat, add zucchini spirals and cook until tender, approximately 5 minutes. Remove from pan and place in a colander. Press out extra liquid and move back to pan. Add Bolognese sauce and mix together.

Serve with a drizzle of fresh extra-virgin olive oil.

# Tamari Ginger Barbecue Chicken

This is my go-to chicken recipe for summer barbecues. I like to serve it with coleslaw, potato salad, a green salad, and beet salad.

2 whole free-range chickens, butchered into 4 legs, 4 thighs, and 4 breasts

2 cups wheat-free store-bought tamari

2-inch piece fresh ginger, grated

5 cloves garlic, smashed

About 2–3 hours before cooking: Place chicken in a large bowl. Add enough tamari to barely cover chicken pieces. Add ginger and garlic and stir. Repeat stirring a few times every hour to rotate the chicken in the marinade.

Preheat outdoor grill or grill pan on medium heat. Cook chicken for about 20–30 minutes, rotating each side every 5 minutes until cooked through. Thick breasts and bone-in thighs will take the longest to cook through. Chicken pieces can also be cooked using a roasting pan for 45 minutes in a preheated 375°F oven. Serve with Dr. Linda's Coleslaw (recipe follows.)

## Dr. Linda's Coleslaw

1 medium red or green cabbage, grated

1 medium sweet onion, peeled and grated

2 large carrots, grated

$1/4$–$1/2$ cup extra-virgin olive oil

2–3 tbsp. apple cider vinegar

2–3 tbsp. Homemade Mayonnaise (page 258) (optional)

1 tsp. sea salt, or more to taste

1 tsp. freshly ground black pepper, or more to taste

In a large bowl, mix together cabbage, onion, and carrots and add enough olive oil to moisten the mixture. Add apple cider vinegar and optionally Homemade Mayonnaise (if using). Season with sea salt and black pepper to taste. Mix thoroughly to flavor and coat all vegetables. Serve chilled.

# SOUTHWEST FIESTA

In the Southwest, we like to eat "family style" at the table, passing around flavorful cooked proteins, beans, guacamole, and salsas, served with fresh corn tortillas and fresh-chopped veggie garnishes to make tacos and burritos. During strict cleansing, you can enjoy a similar experience by serving chili-spiked proteins or vegetables over shredded lettuce as a fiesta salad. During modified cleansing, you may use soft corn tortillas—avoiding the fried, hard-shell kind. (Chewing the soft kind stimulates better digestion.) Serve with a salsa (pages 260–261) and a guacamole (pages 262–263), and have fun using raw jicama as your chip and endive as your scoop.

## Southwest Dry Rub

This rub can be used when grilling meat, poultry, or fish to help develop flavor for your Southwest Fiesta.

2 tsp. sea salt

2 tsp. sweet paprika

1 tsp. granulated garlic

1 tsp. freshly ground black pepper

1 tsp. ground cumin

1 tsp. Mexican oregano, dried

Pinch ground cayenne pepper

Mix all ingredients together in a bowl and pour into a spice shaker. Dry-rub onto your protein of choice right before grilling.

# Grilled Fish

When grilling fish, you want to use a firm fish that will hold up to flipping on the grill.

2–4 portions mahimahi, red snapper, or salmon steak

2–4 tbsp. Southwest Dry Rub (page 254)

1 tbsp. grapeseed oil

1 lime, cut into wedges

Preheat outdoor or stovetop grill pan to medium heat. Rinse the fish in fresh cold water and pat dry. Sprinkle Southwest Dry Rub over both sides of the fish. Brush a small amount of grapeseed oil onto the grill before cooking. Cook the fish for about 5–7 minutes on each side, or until cooked through. Serve with lime wedges.

# Grilled Chicken Fajitas

4 boneless, skinless chicken breasts

4–6 tbsp. Southwest Dry Rub (page 254)

1 tbsp. grapeseed oil

Preheat outdoor or stovetop grill pan to medium heat. On a cutting board, clean the chicken breasts and cut each breast into about 4–5 small to medium-sized pieces. As with chicken paillard, pound out the boneless chicken breasts until thin and tender: Place each piece in a separate ziplock or other plastic bag and pound with the flat side of a meat tenderizer, a mallet, or a rolling pin. Sprinkle a generous amount of Southwest Dry Rub on each side of the breasts. Brush a small amount of grapeseed oil on the grill before cooking. Grill breasts 4–5 minutes on each side until cooked through. Slice and serve as part of your Southwest Fiesta with Fajita Veggies (recipe follows), a salsa (pages 260–261), a guacamole (pages 262–263), garnishes, and tortillas (optional).

## Fajita Veggies

2 bell peppers, sliced into strips

1 sweet onion, cut into half-inch-thick half rounds

2–4 pattypan squashes, quartered

1 zucchini or yellow squash, diced

8–10 baby carrots, halved

1 tbsp. grapeseed oil

Juice of 2 limes

1 tbsp. Southwest Dry Rub (page 254)

Heat a cast-iron skillet at medium heat on the grill or stovetop. Add all veggies and grapeseed oil, moving them around the pan occasionally. Halfway through cooking, add lime juice and the Southwest Dry Rub. More lime can be added to taste. Cook until a nice char is visible and vegetables are tender.

## Garnish (for Proteins and/or Vegetables)

1 head romaine or butter lettuce, shredded (if serving chicken, meat, or vegetables) or 1/2 purple cabbage, shredded (if serving fish)

2 fresh tomatoes, diced

1/2 cup fresh cilantro, finely minced

1 large English cucumber, diced

1 lime, cut into wedges

2 cups home-cooked black beans from Cuban Black Bean Soup (page 228)

Salsa Fresca/Pico de Gallo (page 260)

Tomatillo Salsa Fresca (page 261)

Traditional Guacamole (page 262) or Garden Herb Guacamole (page 263)

Soft organic corn tortillas (optional)

Present each garnish in an individual bowl or all of them together on a large cutting board. Serve family style to accompany Fajita Veggies (above), Grilled Chicken Fajitas (page 255), or Grilled Fish (page 255).

## Poached Fish Fillets

A delicately prepared fresh fish is a good choice for a simple protein meal.

2 medium onions

2 medium carrots

1 stalk celery

8–10 parsley stems

2 tbsp. butter

$1/2$ bay leaf

$1/4$ tsp. tarragon

$1/8$ tsp. sea salt

Freshly ground black pepper

$1/4$ lb. fresh mushrooms, diced

8 fillets of wild fish, such as salmon, branzino, or sea bass

Sea salt and fresh ground black pepper to taste

1 cup dry white French vermouth or apple cider vinegar

Cut the onions, carrots, celery, and parsley in the finest possible dice, and cook over low heat with butter, bay leaf, tarragon, sea salt, and pinch of freshly ground black pepper, simmering for 20 minutes. Add fresh mushrooms and cook for another 10 minutes.

Use a sharp knife to score each fish fillet on the side that was closest to the skin, lightly making a few diagonal cuts to prevent fillets from curling up during cooking.

Lightly salt and pepper fish. Place a spoonful of cooked vegetable mixture over half the fish, then fold over the other half on top, and arrange fillets in a buttered baking dish.

Pour vermouth over fillets, and enough water to cover the fish halfway. Set in 375°F oven for about 15–20 minutes or until the fish flakes easily.

# DRESSINGS, DIPS, AND CONDIMENTS

Use these any way you like to enhance your simple meals—drizzled onto salads or cooked vegetables, as dips for crudités, or on top of your cooked proteins.

## Simple French Dressing

1 cup extra-virgin olive oil

$^1/_8$ cup lemon juice

1 tsp. vegetable seasoning such as Herbamare

1 tsp. honey

Blend or whisk all ingredients until smooth. Store in a tightly sealed glass jar in the refrigerator; keeps for up to one week.

## Homemade Mayonnaise

Fresh homemade mayonnaise or aioli is delicious over steamed fish or steamed vegetables, as a salad dressing, or as a dip for steamed artichokes.

4 egg yolks

2 tsp. Dijon mustard

Juice of 1 lemon

3 oz. water

4 cups extra-virgin olive oil

Sea salt to taste

Fresh ground white pepper to taste

Place egg yolks, mustard, lemon juice, and water in blender or food processor. Begin blending. Drip olive oil in slowly, drop by drop, until mixture starts to thicken. Increase olive oil stream gradually until all oil has been worked in. Add salt and white pepper to taste. Store in a tightly sealed glass jar in the refrigerator; keeps for up to one week.

## Aioli

2 cloves garlic

1 large egg yolk

2 tsp. fresh lemon juice

$1/2$ tsp. Dijon mustard

$1/4$ cup extra-virgin olive oil

3 tbsp. vegetable oil

Sea salt and fresh ground black pepper to taste

Mince and mash garlic to a paste with a pinch of salt, using a large, heavy knife or a mortar and pestle. Whisk together egg yolk, lemon juice, and mustard in a bowl. In separate bowl, combine oils; add them to yolk mixture a few drops at a time, whisking constantly, until all oil is incorporated and mixture is emulsified.

Whisk in garlic paste and season with salt and pepper.

Store in a tightly sealed glass jar in the refrigerator; keeps for up to one week.


## Jalapeño Sauce

This is almost always ready to go in my refrigerator, to accompany grilled vegetables, hummus, or grilled Lebanese-Style Marinated Grilled Chicken (page 250).

10 jalapeño peppers, cored and chopped

2 cloves garlic, peeled and chopped

4 tbsp. extra-virgin olive oil

Juice of 2 lemons

1–2 tsp. sea salt

Place all ingredients in blender or food processor. Blend for 3–5 minutes until smooth. Note that jalapeños tend to vary in spice and flavor. Because of this, always taste the sauce after blending. Sometimes more lemon, more salt, more olive oil, or even some jalapeño membrane can be added to adjust flavor to your taste. Beware this is a spicy sauce!

## Salsa de Agua Chile

I learned about this salsa during one of my trips down to Mexico. This is a salsa version of the flavors that make up the spicy marinade for mexican ceviche. It goes great with most seafood. Use caution when preparing and eating serrano chilies, as they can be very spicy!

1 cup roughly chopped celery stalks

1 cup loosely chopped cucumber

½ small red onion, chopped

½ cup fresh cilantro, packed

Juice of 3–4 limes

1–2 serrano chili peppers, cored and chopped (see note below)

1 tsp. or more of sea salt to taste

Place all ingredients in blender or food processor. Blend for 3–5 minutes until smooth.

**NOTE:** When preparing serrano chilies, wear gloves and wash hands and surfaces immediately afterward.

## Salsa Fresca/Pico de Gallo

Every May at Light Harmonics we plant our summer garden, replete with squashes, cucumbers, beans, peppers, greens, herbs, tomatillos, and heirloom tomatoes. Summertime means a bounty of fresh produce and of course delicious vine-ripened tomatoes. Using these ingredients to make a quick, fresh garden salsa is something we do weekly during the summer.

2 medium fresh tomatoes, deseeded and finely diced

⅓–½ cup fresh cilantro

½ red or white onion, finely diced

2 jalapeños, deseeded and finely diced

Juice of 1–2 limes

½ tsp. sea salt, or more to taste

Place all ingredients in a mixing bowl and combine. This salsa is best eaten right away but should last covered in the refrigerator for at least 1 week.

## Tomatillo Salsa Fresca

Tomatillos are very common in Mexican cuisine and can be found at many supermarkets or Latin markets, usually close to the jalapeños. I grow them every
year in my summer garden, along with cilantro and jalapeños.

**8–10 tomatillos, husks removed,
chopped**

**$1/3$–$1/2$ cup fresh cilantro**

**2 cloves garlic, peeled and chopped**

**2 jalapeños, deseeded and chopped**

**Juice of 1–2 limes**

**$1/2$ tsp. sea salt, or more to taste**

Place all ingredients in blender or food processor. Blend for 3–5 minutes until
smooth. If the salsa is too watery, the mixture can be strained. You can save the
tomatillo water, which can be used as a marinade or combined with olive oil to
make a salad dressing.

## Homemade Hummus

It is convenient to have homemade hummus ready for the family, after school
as a healthy snack or as part of a mediterranean meal.

**$1^1/2$ cups garbanzo beans, drained
and fully cooked ($3/4$ cup dried yields
about $1^1/2$ cups)**

**2–3 tbsp. tahini**

**2 cloves garlic, peeled and chopped**

**1 tbsp. ground cumin**

**Juice of 1 lemon**

**Sea salt and freshly ground black
pepper to taste**

**$1/2$ cup extra-virgin olive oil**

**1 jalapeño, deseeded and diced
(optional)**

Place all ingredients in a food processor except olive oil and jalapeño. Begin
blending, allowing ingredients to mix and become smooth. While processing
you can remove the top center lid, opening up the feeder tube. I like to slowly
add olive oil through the feeder tube, which helps the consistency to become
velvety smooth and rich with olive-oil flavor. The diced jalapeño can be optionally added at the end to make a spicy hummus.

## Guacamole Two Ways

We try to have avocados on hand for slicing on top of a grain or a salad or for a quick guacamole to stir up for fun! When making guacamole for a group, consider one small-medium avocado per person. You don't want to make too much extra guacamole, since avocados quickly oxidize and do not last much longer than a day or two.

### Traditional Guacamole

4 avocados, pits and peels removed

$1/3$ cup cilantro, finely chopped

Juice of 2 limes

1 tsp. ground cumin

1 tbsp. finely diced fresh garlic

1 tsp. sea salt, or more to taste

1–2 small jalapeños, finely diced

1 cup romaine lettuce, washed and shredded

$1/2$ jicama, peeled and thinly sliced

2 carrots, thinly sliced diagonally

$1/2$ large English cucumber, thinly sliced diagonally

Use a fork to mash together avocados, cilantro, lime juice, cumin, garlic, sea salt, and diced jalapeños in a mixing bowl. Taste and add more salt or lime as desired. Remove from bowl and serve on a nest of shredded lettuce with jicama, carrots, and cucumber used as "chips."

## Garden Herb Guacamole

4 avocados, pits and peels removed

$1/4$ sweet onion, finely diced

1 clove garlic, peeled and minced

Dash ground cumin

Juice of 1 lemon

1 tsp. sea salt, or more to taste

$1/4$ cup cilantro, finely chopped

$1/4$ cup mint or tarragon, finely chopped

$1/4$ cup flat-leaf parsley, finely chopped

$1/4$ cup fresh basil, finely chopped

$1/2$ jicama, peeled and thinly sliced

2 carrots, thinly sliced diagonally

$1/2$ large English cucumber, thinly sliced diagonally

Use a fork to mash together avocados, onion, garlic, cumin, lemon juice, and sea salt in a mixing bowl. Once smooth, stir in cilantro, mint, parsley, and basil. Taste and add more salt or lemon as desired. Remove from bowl and serve with jicama, carrots, and cucumber as "chips."

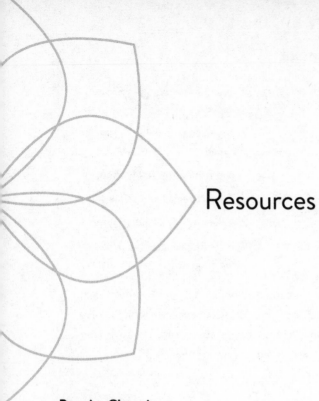

# Resources

## Parasite Cleansing

### Lab Elymental's The Milk Cleanse
Eight-day Milk Cleanse using all natural herbs to support detoxification of parasites.
*A percentage of proceeds of this product goes toward research in Lyme Disease and other tick-borne illnesses.
www.themilkcleanse.com

### UNIKEY HEALTH—My Colon Cleansing Kit
Intestinal parasite cleanse for micro organisms detoxification support.
www.unikeyhealth.com

### Advance Naturals—ParaMax Cleanse
ParaMax provides natural support to assist with the detoxification of parasites in the intestines.
www.advancednaturals.com

## Books on Homeopathy

*Homeopathic Medicine at Home: Natural Remedies for Everyday Ailments and Minor Injuries* by Maesimund B. Panos, MD

*Homeopathic Self-Care: The Quick and Easy Guide for the Whole Family* by Robert Ullman

## For Advanced Reading

*The Science of Homeopathy* by George Vithoulkas

*Magic of the Minimum Dose* by Dr. Dorothy Shepherd

*The Patient, Not the Cure* by Margery G. Blackie

*The Organon of Medicine* by Samuel Hahnemann

## Homeopathic Remedies

Most health food stores carry homeopathic remedies. The following are companies that offer remedies by shipment if unavailable locally.

www.boironusa.com
www.hylands.com
www.homeopathyworks.com

For the Original Bach Flower Remedies including Rescue Remedy
www.bachflower.com

## Books on Radionics and Radiesthesia

*Radionics and the Subtle Anatomy of Man* by David Tansley

*Principles and Practice of Radiesthesia* by Abbe Mermet

*The Patterns of Health* by Aubrey Westlake

## For Information on Radionics, Radiesthesia, and Dowsing

**USPA United States Psychotronics Association**
www.psychotronics.com

**The American Society for Dowsers**
www.dowsers.org

**The Radionic Association UK**
www.radionics.co.uk

**The British Society of Dowsers**
www.BritishDowsers.org

## For Information about Integrative Medicine:

**Global Foundation for Integrative Medicine (GFIM)**
Founded by Dr. Linda Lancaster, GFIM is a 501c nonprofit organization that promotes public awareness, education, and scientific research in the field of Integrative Medicines. For more information visit: www.gfimusa.com

## For Training in Homeopathy, Radiesthesia, and Radionics:

**Light Harmonics Institute**
www.lightharmonics.com

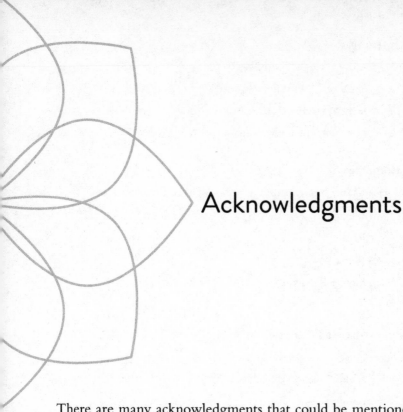

# Acknowledgments

There are many acknowledgments that could be mentioned here. Be it known, that without my patients, students, friends, and family this book could not have been written.

I am most thankful to my son Dr. John Sherdon for being by my side throughout my years of practice, as a son, a student, and as a doctor of Oriental Medicine and subtle medicines at Light Harmonics clinic.

Thank you to all the students of Light Harmonics Institute. A special thank you to Marissa Cascarilla for helping with editing and questioning, where further explanations were needed. To Beatrice Tosti for her inspiration and love of cooking we share, to graduate students of Light Harmonics, Lonnie Jelinek and Aimee Whalen for continuing on the path of healing, and to Taya Thurman, for encouraging me to write a book many years before. I am also grateful for my friend, Lutie Larsen, who I share the love of radionics with.

Thank you to my visionary friend, Beth Rosenthal, who *demanded* I write a book and graciously introduced me to my agents, Steve Troha and Dado Derviskadic, who proclaimed "don't you want to write down what your bedrock is?" It rung a bell and here we are.

And thank you to Amely Greeven, a health writer, patient, and student of Light Harmonics, who helped me write this book and *softened* the scientific language for better understanding. In the year 2000, Amely interviewed me for a prominent women's magazine about Naturopathy, and I told her that one day I would ask her to help me write a book explaining the subtle fields of medicine. She agreed almost 20 years later.

A special thank you to Alyse Diamond, my editor, who I count on for guidance and knowing what the reader wants to know.

And last, but not least, thank you to my partner Ken Diehl for supporting me throughout the process of writing this book and for sharing in our healthy lifestyle together.

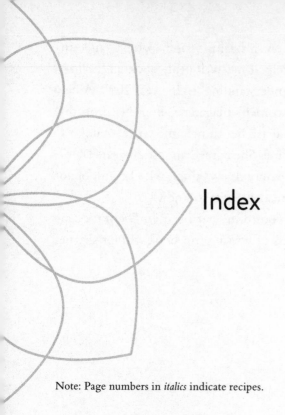

# Index

Note: Page numbers in *italics* indicate recipes.

fats
- carbohydrate consumption and, 96–98
- liver and, 95–96
- nuts affecting liver, 99
- oils, 136–137, 143, 171, 195
- refined, high-temperature cooking and, 95–96

five elements
- about: overview and combinations of, 22–23
- digestive fire and, xix, 22, 32, 81, 85–87, 174
- etheric field and, 22–23
- five parasites, five passions and, 66–74

food. See also Liver-Cleansing Program; specific main ingredients
- about: overview of sacred power of, 104–105
- attitude and timing of eating, 121–125, 149–150
- author's background with, xviii–xix
- biodynamic, 110–111, 134
- blessing, 145
- case studies, 114–115, 124–125
- cleansing (Clorox Food Bath), 112, 115, 144–145
- combining, 119–120, 147–148
- conscious connection to eating, 105
- conscious nutrition guidelines, 115–125
- discovering unseen energy of, 107–108
- etheric energy from, 19–20, 110–111
- honoring the act of eating, 121–125
- incoherent energy patterns from, 111–112
- kitchen equipment to cook, 200–201
- liver's clock and, 122
- locally produced, 115–116
- love and, 187
- meat and vegetables, 117
- minerals and, 108–109
- modern conundrum, 112–115
- natural laws and, 113–114
- optimal energy from, 111
- organic, 19–20, 98, 110–111, 113, 115–116, 141
- pantry items, 189–200
- peace and, 123–124
- preparing, xviii–xix, xx, 120–121, 148, 187–189, 201–209
- resonance effect and, 19–20
- seasonal eating, 118–119
- soil and energetics of, 109–112
- subtle nature and power of, xix, 105–107, 110–112

- traditional health care practices and, 21–22
- unhealthy, purging from kitchen, 189
- vegetable and fruit importance, 116–117

frequency, laws of, 32–35
fried foods, 136

fruit
- cleansing, 144–145
- combining, 142–143, 147–148
- 80:20 ratio of plant to protein intake, 146–147
- to enjoy on diet, 142
- importance of vegetables and, 116–117
- seasonal, 118–119, 142, 190
- shopping for, 189–190
- to stock, 190–191

giardia, 52, 53–54, 57
grains, 137–138, 156–158, 161, 196, 207. See also rice
green beans, 202, 208, 225, 230, 238
greens, 193, 217, 226, 227. See also kale; salads
grilling, 205–206
gunas (sattva, rajas, tamas), 91

Hahnemann, Samuel, 12. See also Organon of Medicine (Hahnemann)

Harmonic Healing
- about: overview of, xxv–xxvi; using this book for, xxvii–xxix, 6–8
- author's journey to discovering, xvii–xxvi
- knowledge of masters infused in, xx–xxv. See also Bhattacharya, Dr. A. K.; Jayasuriya, Professor Anton; Parcells, Dr. Hazel; Yogi Bhajan (Yogi Ji)
- medicines used in, xxvi
- principles (five) of, xxx
- resonance effect and, 19–20
- what you can gain from, xxvii–xxix

harmony, living in, 75–76
harmony of energy patterns, 19–20, 25–26, 33

headaches, liver cleanse and, 168

health and healing. See also balance
- connecting invisible dimensions of, 125–126
- disconnects between physical and subtle bodies and, 81–82
- forces challenging, 2–3
- hidden key to, 1. See also etheric energy
- interferences with. See interferences

*About the Author*

DR. LINDA LANCASTER is a Naturopathic and Homeopathic physician. In 1987, she founded Light Harmonics Institute, an energy medicine clinic and educational center based in Santa Fe, New Mexico. Her training includes Ayurveda, yoga, medical radiesthesia, radionics, subtle energy healing, counseling, nutrition, herbal medicine, and detoxification methods. Her life-changing health and cleansing programs have been offered to her patients and their families for nearly forty years.